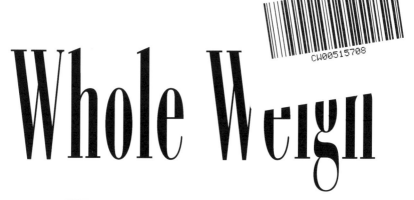

Whole Weigh

How to Quit Dieting and Start Living a Healthy and Whole Life.

Charlotte Denny Henley

Chagoh Publications
Huron, SD

Quotes with Illustrations
Paul Libeau and Barry Trower
P.S.A.Ventures
London, ON Canada

Copyright © 2012 by Charlotte Denny Henley
Published by Chagoh Publications, Huron, SD

For information contact info@wholeweigh.com

ISBN-10: 0985376007
ISBN-13: 978-0985376000

First Edition, Revised

Dedication

* * *

This book is dedicated to the memory of my sister
Kathleen Friedrich who was blessed with incredible insights
and a passion for truth, and to the memory of my mother
Mary for her joyful enthusiasm for life and living.

Table of Conents

Appendices

Introduction

"Frequent dieting is perhaps the single best predictor of future weight gain."

The Obesity Myth, Paul Campos[1]

You have picked up this book hoping for the solution to your weight problem. Well, let me say up front, I'm not promising a ten-pound weight loss in two weeks or the best fat-burning exercise routine. What I do offer you is a gentle journey intended to bring peace of mind to your relationship with food, diet, exercise, and your body. You may lose weight on this journey, but the health of your body, mind and spirit is the focus. *Whole Weigh* will open doors to a new way of thinking about you, your body, food, and exercise. You were attracted to this book because you're ready.

I felt compelled to write this book because of my personal experience with diets. Having been down that road many times, I know the diet cycle is painful and frustrating. I suspect you've done the same thing. Read on and see if the journey sounds familiar.

You buy a book or product, burst out of the starting blocks with enthusiasm, and within a few days you stumble. You fight with yourself and make several attempts to get back on track. Perhaps you stick it out for several weeks or months and manage to lose weight. Then one day, without realizing it, you're no longer on a diet. The pounds creep back on and within months you've ballooned back up. You torture yourself about your lack of self-control. You avoid thinking about it, but are reminded each day when you stand in front of your closet and agonize. Nothing fits. In an effort to find some inner peace, you try to convince yourself that you are okay just the way you are, but deep down you're tortured.

When a new diet comes along, you swallow your pride and try again. "I've got to do it this time." But a little voice, we'll call your

---

1 Campos, Paul. 2004. The Obesity Myth: Why America's Obsession with Weight Is Hazardous to Your Health. New York: Gotham Books, p. xxii.

inner critic, spreads a message to your brain cells, and you listen. "Go ahead and try another diet. You've tried so many times and have always failed. You know you can't stay on a diet." This inner voice will sabotage any forward progress.

You desperately try to stick to the diet despite the message from your inner critic. When you abandon the diet, you have to bear the shame. You're embarrassed and wonder what everybody's thinking. Your inner critic will triumphantly announce, "See? I told you. You're fat and a failure." Depressed, frustrated, and anguished, you give up, until some new diet tempts you with promises of quick results. All you need to do is diet and exercise according to the plan, and you'll lose weight. You are tempted once again. You have no other options. The inner critic salivates, gets ready, and takes aim. I know this story well because it is mine.

The inner critic, of course, is the negative chanting in your head cultivated by life's experiences. Certainly the accumulation of diet failures generates lots of negative material on which the inner critic can feed. But you also have an inner champion that roots for you and gets you to believe there is nothing you can't do. What if we fed the inner champ so it would grow strong and become the dominant voice in your head? *Whole Weigh* does just that—it feeds the inner champ and builds internal strength. I believe you have to feel good about yourself to make a change. Diets make you feel bad.

My Story

I was an active child growing up in Silver Lake, Wisconsin and Queens, New York. I was physically gifted, so I could easily run, swim, play stickball, and dance. I took professional dance classes at the June Taylor School of Dance, with a dream of being a New York City Rockette. But at the age of twelve I started to notice I had thick thighs compared to the other dancers at the school. I was fixated on every dancer's thighs on TV and in Broadway shows, looking for the one gal that had thighs like mine, and all I saw were long lean legs. In my mind, the writing was on the wall: you can't be a dancer with big thighs. So, the dream died.

As I became a young adult I used my physical abilities to play sports and dabble with running. I was fairly free of the idea of losing weight, but I still had a thing about my thighs. I married young, moved to Canada, and gave birth to two sons. There was no abnormal weight gain during pregnancy, just a few stretch marks; it was still all about my thighs.

My marriage ended when my boys were still young. At the time, I lived in the small town of Grimsby, Ontario, and was employed as a waitress at a steak house. One day, at the encouragement of my friend Gloria, I pitched an idea to the Parks and Recreation Department. It was for an innovative fitness program for women, called Fitness in the Park. We used the outdoor exercise stations in the park and experimented with many different types of activities including, hiking, lawn bowling, badminton, and cycling in the summer; curling, snow shoeing, skating and cross country skiing in the winter. The program was a huge success, but my body or more specifically, my thighs, were now "out there."

I was in a business where body shape mattered, an idea I conjured up in my own mind. To me, my thighs were a liability. My solution was to lose weight, even though I weighed only 125 pounds at the time. Now, of course, I recognize that losing weight was not going to change the shape of my body, which was gifted to me at my conception.

I went back to college as a mature student and majored in physical education. In the first year of my degree program, I was asked to become a trainer for Fitness Ontario. It was a great opportunity but I had to be convinced I was worthy. I didn't have a degree like all the other trainers, and secretly I wondered if they noticed my body shape—my big thighs. How would I compare to the really thin trainers? It all seems so ridiculous, as I tell this story. I was fit, healthy and 125 pounds. Despite my insecurities, I did accept the invitation and became a fitness leadership trainer, so the war with my thighs began in earnest.

During this time, I was teaching up to fourteen hours of fitness classes and running ten miles a week, plus teaching folk dance at my alma mater. I was incredibly fit, but that didn't stop my inner critic: "You're not a credible fitness trainer with those thighs. You look fat." I nursed this attitude despite my popularity as a trainer and leader.

I tried all the fad diets that came along, and like most of you I would lose weight and gain it back, plus a few extra pounds. My clothes and fitness apparel were carefully selected to cover my hips and thighs. I always felt very self-conscious; I never felt as credible as I thought the other trainers were. I look back now and realize how this attitude infiltrated my professional life in fitness. I was a competent and enthusiastic trainer, shadowed by my negative body image. I allowed many opportunities to pass me by in order to satisfy my inner critic, even the possibility of an exercise TV show. My body shape determined my sense of worth as a fitness trainer.

Once I moved to South Dakota in my late forties, I was incognito. I felt relieved as my weight crept over 180 pounds. Now I could just be me, and not carry the burden of being a fitness professional. I had escaped my self-imposed prison. How silly, but I truly felt that way.

My escape was short lived because I had to depend on my degree and past work experience for employment. In time, I carefully reconstructed my inner prison: I'm fat and therefore I have limited credibility as a fitness trainer, physical education professor, or fitness business owner. I taught courses and classes with enthusiasm and wisdom, but I secretly held on to silly notions that I was constantly being judged. My own thoughts created the mess inside my head, because my students and colleagues offered me nothing but respect.

As the years passed I dieted more and gained more, nearing 200 pounds. Most days began with a promise to myself.

"This will be a no sugar day."

"I'll just have soup for lunch, nothing else."

"I'll walk during my lunch hour."

"I'm starting my diet today and this time I'm sticking to it."

It was a constant barrage of promises made and promises broken.

Diet Free Declaration Day

Then one day I gave it up. I stopped dieting and stopped weighing. The idea of wasting so much mental and physical energy on my body image suddenly seemed so absurd. I was sick of waking up to the burden of another day on a diet. I was emotionally spent and diet fatigued. I couldn't do it anymore. I had tempered my career to wait for the day I would be thin. It wasn't going to happen. My life could not unfold and expand as long as I was wrestling with my body.

The moment I said, "I'm done," I was free. Years of accumulated anguish left me. I could instantly sense I was travelling down a different road. There was still work to be done, but I was free. My inner critic could no longer badger me about dieting.

Now, my internal work revolved around self-acceptance. I had to learn to love myself and my body in a whole new way. My attention sifted from what was wrong with my body and my life to what was right. My inner critic had lost the center stage.

Since giving up dieting, my body weighs less, not a lot, but definitely less. I've stabilized my weight without any restrained eating or extraordinary exercise regime. Now, health and personal achievements are my goals. I am diet free, healthy, happy, and living a whole life.

Strengthening My Convictions

I have always believed you need to live life in harmony with Mother Nature, so I eat organic food whenever possible, and never trust any medical solution that doesn't respect the nature of the body. I'm also suspicious of any shoe or apparatus that alters the natural function of the body. I really trust God's design.

Physical activity needs to be fun and playful, not a chore. In service to my clients, I discourage dieting and teach them to respect their unique physical characteristics and capabilities. Too bad I didn't follow my own advice whenever I felt the urge to diet.

In my professional career, I have taught hundreds of aerobic classes, trained hundreds of fitness leaders, and prepared university physical education students to be great champions of quality physical education. I did this in ways that emphasized a playful approach to physical activity, the goodness of fresh foods, and a deep respect for the wisdom of our bodies.

The clarity of my beliefs came into focus once I was an owner of an express fitness center, called the Body Garden. For five years, I interacted daily with chronic dieters. I listened to them and learned about their frustration and agony, which I knew all too well from my own experiences. Their stories revealed the grip body image and weight had on their sense of worth and their ability to live a full life. It was a reflection of my own agony.

I would coach my members to adopt three simple principles for good health: eat close to Mother Nature, go outside and play, and think good thoughts. But I never had a systematic way to teach them how to free themselves from dieting and adopt simple holistic principles for health. They had become accustomed to following a diet plan, and I was only offering guidelines. It was hard for most to make the leap from a specific plan to guiding principles. Over time, I developed a program that people enjoyed, and with that came encouragement to write a book, something I had always wanted to do.

The Tragedy of the War on Obesity

As I write this book, modern industrialized countries around the world are faced with an obesity epidemic as declared by the World Health Organization, the Center for Disease Control and other nations around the world. The war against fat has begun. The United States has one of the highest rates of obesity compared to other countries, and the federal government is mounting an attack. Their intentions are good, but I'm afraid the methods that government institutions and health organizations will use to eradicate human fat will spawn a new generation of eating disorders. We'll evaluate every morsel of food, diet-talk will dominate mealtime discussions, and the diet police will ban substances that make you fat. Your children will get grades on their fatness and thinness, and moral judgments about fat people will increase. Fear of fat will reside deep within our psyches. Self-hatred, shame, guilt, and ridicule will reign. These strategies will generate very deep personal wounds, people will feel lousy, and change will become harder. People may get thin, but they will be deeply wounded.

In contrast, *Whole Weigh* will feed your inner champion so your spirit will grow strong, and you will feel good. Your preoccupation about your body and weight will be diminished by focusing on all the dimensions that make you a vital, unique and magnificent human being. You are more than your physical dimension. You are a bright, loving, intelligent, and gifted being with a great capacity for living a whole, healthy and happy life.

The goal of *Whole Weigh* is to get you feeling good about yourself and to cultivate a harmonious relationship with your body, food, and physical activity. Health, vitality and a zest for living are the outcomes. I can't guarantee that you will lose weight from the wisdom of this book; it's possible, but first, you must be willing to fall in love with yourself and your body. Only then can real behavior change erupt. Health is an expression of your inner self.

So let me make this clear, this is not a weight loss book; it's a holistic health and wellness book for those who have tried and failed numerous times to lose weight. Your inner spirit needs some tender loving care. When you feel good about yourself, your body will respond with glowing health, and your mind will be free to dream.

Something to Think About

What does your inner critic say when you start a new diet? Do you believe you will be successful or do you have doubts? What messages do you tell yourself about your body and weight? How much time do you spend thinking about weight, food, diet and exercise?

PART I

Chronic Dieters
Set Yourselves Free

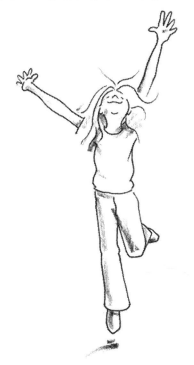

To love
is to set ourselves and others
FREE

Chapter 1

Is The Problem You or the Diet?

"Insanity: Doing the same thing over and over again and expecting different results."

– Albert Einstein

Are you a chronic dieter? Have you been on more than one diet in the past year? Have you tried many different diets in your lifetime, but gain back the weight? Do you drive yourself crazy thinking about and planning the next diet?

Dieters have a failure rate as high as 90%; we take it off, but put it back on. Is it the dieter or the diet that's the problem? It's time to ask that question. When so many of us try so hard, so many times, and fail, maybe diets and dieting are the real problem.

For a moment, think about a diet as any other product or service you purchase. A prescription drug with a 90% failure rate wouldn't get near the marketplace. Imagine a medical procedure that was only successful 10% of the time or a computer that failed to function 90% of the time. You'd never consider purchasing anything with such an outrageous failure rate. But, you keep trying another diet product or program, which produces the same result—take the weight off and put it back on. You blame yourself for the failure, but could you be relying on a faulty product to lose weight? Could the conventional diet template be the primary contributing factor to your failure?

If you're a chronic dieter then you know you're always on the lookout for a different diet—one that will finally take the weight off for good. Let me make this clear: there are no new diets! They are all the same. All diets use the same diet template. Whether high protein, low fat, calorie reduced, low carb, or sugar busting—they're all the same. Every diet scheme requires you to eliminate bad foods, add good foods, count grams, calories or points, drink water, and exercise. You set reasonable goals, journal your food intake, and weigh yourself each week to monitor your progress. There may be slight variations, but the general requirements are the same. At this point you may be wondering how this book could offer you anything different. Is there another template? Yes! Stick with me.

The belief system that shapes the standard diet template is based on three things: one, a scientific-mechanistic model that relates to the body as a machine; two, a type of psychology called behaviorism (known to the general population as behavior modification); and three, the view that the body, mind, and soul are separate from each other.

Jon Robison and Karen Carrier have written a brilliant book for practitioners titled, *The Spirit and Science of Holistic Health,* which outlines the development and influence of these three factors on modern societies' approach to human health. They refer to it as "biomedicine" and explain it this way: "…biomedicine views human beings basically as sophisticated machines that can be analyzed in terms of their parts. Sickness and disease are considered to be malfunctions of the biological mechanisms of the machine."[2] Do you sense the problem here? Stripped away from this belief is the interconnected relationship of the body, mind, and spirit— a grave error in thinking. We are not machines. We are energy; adapting, changing, sensing, feeling and expressing all the dimensions of our human experience.

The biomedical model ignores the interconnectedness of body, mind, and spirit, and instead considers only the body and its individual parts. That is why obesity is considered merely a math problem—too many calories in and not enough burned off. Simply reduce calories and fat grams and increase physical activity and one will reduce body weight and disease risk factors. You can see why the biomedical model is popular and enduring—it's systematic, observable, and easy to measure.

It all seems to make sense, but it doesn't work. The dismal failure rate of losing and maintaining weight loss is enough evidence to scrap the conventional diet template and look around for something new.

---

2 Robison, Jon, and Carrier, Karen. 2004. The Spirit and Science of Holistic Health. Indiana: Author House. p. 32.

Health versus Weight

As I write this book, there is a non-diet movement evolving that promotes intuitive eating and/or spiritual fulfillment as alternative strategies to managing weight. Whole Weigh is part of the movement. Some practitioners in the movement still promote weight loss as the primary goal, while others promote health as the true goal. This leads to some clear differences in approach.

Linda Bacon and Lucy Aphramor, in an article titled "Weight Science: Evaluating the Evidence for a Paradigm Shift," published in *Nutrition Journal* in January 2011, outline the reasons to shift from the diet and weight paradigm to a more holistic health model. The article establishes the high failure rate of dieting and punctuates the additional negative health outcomes of chronic dieting, or what they refer to as *weight cycling.*

The article presents evidence that suggests chronic dieting and not total body weight is more likely to cause high blood pressure, high cholesterol, and insulin resistance—a precursor to diabetes. More importantly, the article establishes that chronic dieting reduces self-esteem and increases the incidence of eating disorders, psychological stress and body dissatisfaction. Negative psychological factors lead to lower levels of physical activity and increased caloric intake. It's not extra weight that causes health problems; it's more likely chronic dieting.[3] Are you starting to get the picture? Dieting has a negative impact on your goal to lose weight and get healthy.

Steven Blair, a champion of *health fitness,* is a former Director of Cooper Aerobics Institute and now a professor at University of South Carolina. He's an all-star researcher on the relationship of health and physical activity. His research reveals that with moderate amounts of physical activity, regardless of your weight, you can be healthy, and in fact you could be healthier than thin people who are physically inactive. Not all thin people are healthy and not all fat people are unhealthy. Blair is the best example of his own findings on health versus weight. He is an avid runner with a short, stocky build. His body mass index (BMI), which uses the

---

3 Bacon, Linda and Aphramor, Lucy. January 24, 2011. Weigh science: evaluating the evidence for a paradigm shift. *Nutrition Journal* 2011, 10:9. Available at www.nutritionj.com/content/10/1/9

relationship of height and weight to determine health risk, is high. He's classified as obese despite his good health and active lifestyle.

This, of course, questions the validity of BMI as a classification tool for health risks related to weight. Currently BMI is used by most medical professionals despite research that suggests it's not as accurate as once thought, but they continue to use it because it's non-invasive and easy. I'm not going to argue about its validity in this book, but I will tell you I'm not a big fan. Too many people are placed in the overweight or obese categories that don't belong, especially those with muscular body types. With or without a muscular body type, you may see yourself as having a normal weight or being slightly overweight, with good health, but your BMI score may classify you as obese, implying you have lots of health risks. That's demoralizing. Common sense needs to prevail.

There are many different body types and many different measurements of health. Weight is not the only determinant of your health, and BMI is a poor indicator of your weight classification and your health. The medical establishment needs more diversity in their assessment tools and broader ranges of interpretation. My advice is to ignore BMI.

If you need more convincing that diets are hazardous and a goal weight is problematic, the books *Health at Every Size,* by Linda Bacon, PhD, *The Obesity Myth,* by Paul Campos, JD, and *Big Fat Lies* by Glenn Gaesser, PhD are loaded with the evidence. Read them all to recognize the futility of dieting and to release any fixation you may have on a goal weight as the predictor of your health. Everyone benefits from good nutrition and physical activity, regardless of size; hence, you can be healthy at any size.

What's a Person to Do?

"But, I want to lose weight." I know that's what you're saying to yourself at this point of the book. You're afraid I am going to suggest you accept your body as it is and be happy, and that is something you cannot imagine. Try imagining this:

 My body is full of energy and it moves with ease. I feel good. I wake in the morning enthused about the dawning of a new day. My health is glowing and my attitude is upbeat. I feel so alive.

Isn't this what you want? If you feel this way does it matter if you're not at your "perfect" weight? You can certainly weigh less, but why drive yourself crazy for five, ten, fifteen or even twenty pounds when you can be healthy, fit and happy whether you're near or far from your goal weight?

You will find, as you read this book, that your goal weight is the primary nemesis of your attempts to lose weight. You can weigh less when you give up dieting, and focus, within a positive framework, on wholesome foods, fun physical activities and good thoughts. And let me remind you, the real problem is not losing weight; it's keeping the weight off. That's the benchmark that produces the 90% failure rates among dieters.

To embark on the journey towards a healthy energized body that moves with ease, you will need to change the way you see yourself. It's self-love and acceptance that prompts good health and positive behaviors, not a calorie reduced diet or any other diet. Weight loss is a likely outcome when you adopt a more holistic approach to health, but you can only get there if you first give up dieting and all the rituals that go with it; second, fall in love with your magnificent self, just the way you are; and third, make health your goal, instead of a goal weight.

The purpose of this book is to persuade you to abandon dieting, and guide you to a more holistic way of relating to yourself, food, physical activity and life. You will benefit by releasing your fixation on weight and diet rituals—all the stuff that drives you crazy. You'll rebuild yourself by connecting to all the dimensions that make you whole, discovering your personal strengths, and generating a clear vision for yourself at your best. This will lead you to a greater sense of peace and harmony, something I believe we all crave. From that place you will be more open and willing to change, and more willing to adopt the three simple principles to better health. They are:

- Eat Close to Mother Nature
- Go Outside and Play
- Think Good Thoughts

When these basic principles are integrated within your body, mind and spirit, your health will flourish. You'll still have to make choices about your behavior and commit to change if you want to weigh less, but you'll do it from a place of self-love and respect and without all the impediments of a traditional diet. This is a much easier road to travel.

Assignment

Get yourself a journal and commit to completing the questions that are presented throughout the book. This will help you increase self-awareness and self-acceptance. This is the true source of a whole, healthy life.

Chapter 2

The Traditional Diet Template: A Prescription for Failure

"Remember the two benefits of failure. First, if you do fail, you learn what doesn't work; and second, the failure gives you the opportunity to try a new approach."

– Roger Von Oech

To begin the Whole Weigh journey, it's helpful to understand the roots of the current diet template so you can move past them and adopt a new way of thinking. There are seven basic premises related to the current diet template. Some have merit and contain elements of truth, but when packaged together they unintentionally sabotage diet success, but more importantly, they distort our relationships with our bodies, food, and exercise.

Let's examine the seven premises that fuel our inner critic and breed negative associations with our bodies, exercise, and food. This, I hope will convince you to give up dieting.

1. The Body Is a Machine: Fix It!
2. The Reason for Living: Avoid Disease
3. Just Twenty-One Days to Change Your Habits
4. It's Simple: Change Your Lifestyle
5. It's Mere Math: Calories In—Calories Out
6. Fear: The Primary Motivator
7. Critical Self-Analysis

1. The Body Is a Machine: Fix It!

The template for most diets begins with the notion that the body is like a machine, made of many individual parts that need maintenance and repair. Knees and hips are mechanical joints we can replace. Your brain can be medicated, blood vessels scraped, and the digestive tract rerouted. X-rays, MRIs, and CAT scans produce pictures of body parts for "mechanics", otherwise known as doctors, to interpret, and drugs target a precise problem, such as cholesterol, blood pressure, heart function, and digestion.

Viewing the body as a machine has triggered remarkable advances in medical diagnosis and treatment. But the application of this viewpoint has a downside. It fails to acknowledge the mysteries of the body and its complex interconnected processes. Treating only one part of the body may throw off the balance in other parts of the body. This viewpoint also fails to consider the contribution of our emotions and spiritual energy to health and healing. Faith, joy, happiness, personal satisfaction, and good relationships are ignored as contributors to health, when in fact these aspects of the human experience contribute significantly to our health and well-being.

In this one-dimensional view, obesity is nothing more than a disease that calls for domination, deprivation, and alteration. Eat fewer calories than you burn. If that doesn't do the trick, then staple your stomach, or suck out the fat. That's what you get when you see the body as a machine: one-dimension; no heart or soul. I know these medical procedures have some great outcomes and psychological support, but the primary premise still remains: you go to war with your body.

Something to Think About

Have you ever considered a medical procedure to help you lose weight? Have you ever taken medication or a commercial remedy to aid weight loss? What were the results? How did you feel? How would you describe your relationship with your body—harmonious or domineering?

---

2. The Reason for Living: Avoid Disease

When you relate to the body as a machine, you focus on the malfunction of the parts and indicators, such as high blood pressure, cholesterol, blood sugar levels, and weight. They say you have to know your medical numbers. The problem is these numbers overtake your life and lifestyle. Controlling your cholesterol, blood sugar and blood pressure becomes the ultimate goal in your life, or so it seems. No one wants his or her body to malfunction, but avoiding disease should not consume our lives. MeMe Roth, founder of the National Action Against Obesity, is the poster spokesperson for this obnoxious way of thinking. Here's the story.

Jordin Sparks was one of the finalists for the 2007 *American Idol* on FOX; a thirteen-week singing competition on TV profiling people in pursuit of their dreams. Jordin was seventeen at the time and bursting with talent. Each week she graciously accepted criticism and praise from the judges and came back stronger the following week. Nearly 50 million people watched each week as her performances and confidence grew. With 72 million votes cast on the final night, Jordin won the competition, and with the utmost humility, thanked her family, her fans, and God. Then with poise beyond her seventeen years, she sang her final song, "This Is My Now." It all felt so good. I was inspired.

This is the phenomenon of *American Idol* and other shows like it; ordinary people taking a chance. When they triumph, they inspire all of us to reach for something more—to believe in ourselves—despite our doubts and fears. Jordin, with grace and humility, was not afraid to grow into her dream in front of America. What a wonderful role model, don't you think?

Well, MeMe Roth the founder of the National Action Against Obesity believed something entirely different. She didn't think Jordin should win the competition because Jordan was "not healthy." She stated on FOX TV's *Neil Cavuto Show*, "When I look at Jordin, I see diabetes, I see heart disease, I see high cholesterol. That's what's so bad about this—she is not the vision of health, she is the vision of unhealth"[4] MeMe Roth may mean well, but she is seriously misguided. MeMe is promoting the idea that weight is the ultimate determinant of our worth. Really? Should thinness be our ultimate goal in life and does weight truly define our health?

---

4 Roth, MeMe. Appeared on the Neil Cavuto Show, May 23, 2007, Fox News.

Let's get this straight. Evidence shows that weight does not necessarily determine health. In fact, the research led by Stephen Blair while at the Cooper Aerobics Institute indicates, that overweight people who are physically active may be considered healthier than inactive thin people. "Thin people do not have a monopoly on health and fitness," states Blair.[5] Thin bodies can indicate eating disorders, drug abuse, smoking, or malnutrition. The point is, weight does not determine health.

Our health is greatly influenced by our emotional, spiritual, and social well-being. There is plenty of evidence that our thoughts, feelings, and relationships help determine our health, but how do you measure a thought? How do you measure a relationship? How do you measure overcoming fear and winning *American Idol?* You can't, so the mechanics—our doctors and dieticians—disregard what they can't measure and instead fixate on blood pressure, cholesterol, calories, and fat grams, and then assess your health based on these measurements. What we measure becomes the focus of our health and then consumes our lives. People like MeMe Roth, who are crusading against obesity, demonstrate their ignorance of the true meaning of health.

Let me reiterate: avoiding disease is not the reason for living. I suggest our reason for living is to use our God-given talents to positively affect the world. Jordin Sparks, with her beautiful voice, is an expression of a much greater purpose in life than avoiding disease. Her God-given talent—not her weight, nor her cholesterol level—is the source of her self-worth. She inspires me and makes my soul feel good.

Something to Think About

Do you allow your weight to define your self-worth? How often do you talk about weight, cholesterol, and other health measurements? How does that make you feel? What do you believe is the reason for living?

---

5 Gaesser, Glenn A. 2002. Big Fat Lies: The Truth about Your Weight and Your Health. Carlsbad, CA: Gurze. p. xiii.

3. Just Twenty-One Days to Change Your Habits

The claims are all over the bookshelves and Internet: "Change Your Habits in Twenty-One Days." Some even guarantee it! I question the wisdom of this notion. Many people have lost and kept weight off for months and even years, but then suddenly—or gradually—the weight came back. What happened to those good habits? Even being diagnosed with cancer or heart disease is not a reliable motivator to adopt new habits. "Old Habits Die Hard" is a more appropriate claim.

As it turns out, this concept came from Dr. Maxwell Maltz, a plastic surgeon who, through his own experiences and research, promoted the idea of behavior change in just twenty-one days. But those who boast his claim oversimplify the application and fail to understand Dr. Maltz's whole premise.

Dr. Maltz believed that change only happens when one has a strong self-image. He recognized extraneous goals such as weight or cholesterol as being important, but not achieved simply by practicing new behaviors. "Self-image is the cornerstone of all the changes that take place in a person. If one's self-image is unhealthy, or faulty, all of his or her efforts will end in failure."[6] Maltz learned this as a plastic surgeon. He noticed that changing people's physical appearance to be more desirable rarely resulted in a happier person. These patients still found fault with themselves. People can temporarily change behavior and feel good, but according to Maltz, "If your 'inner self' is not equal to your 'outer self,' then you will always revert back."[7] This is a real clue to the 90% failure rate of the diet template.

NBC's TV show, *The Biggest Loser,* demonstrates this principle. Contestants are pushed physically far beyond their perceived limitations—running, hiking, and climbing with their 200–400 pound bodies. The trainers aggressively push their team members to recruit every ounce of energy to complete unbelievable, physically challenging tasks. In the process, some contestants uncap amazing personal strength and experience an enormous sense of accomplishment. "Half the battle is bolstering self-esteem. It's

---

6 Wikepedia. en.wikipedia.org/wiki/Maxwell_Maltz, (Retrieved, October 14, 2008).
7 Self Improvement OnLine. www.selfgrowth.com/experts/maxwell_maltz.html (Retrieved, October 14, 2008).

about feeling better about yourself,"[8] said Bob Harper, one of the trainers.

A few of the former *Biggest Loser* contestants were featured on Oprah's TV talk show. Several regained some weight. From my observation, those that maintained their weight expressed their feelings somewhat differently than those who had regained their weight. The ones who were struggling talked about the diet and exercise regime, and offered reasons for their added weight, while those that had kept the weight off spoke of relationships, their families, and how much they have changed personally—they didn't talk about their exercise routine or diet regimen. You have to change from within to maintain change. So let me put this idea in your head; feeling good about yourself is the true goal, not weight loss. Practicing a behavior for twenty-one days is not a guarantee for permanent weight loss—self-love is the "game changer."

Something to Think About

Does it make sense that feeling good about yourself is the real fuel for change? How would you describe your self-image? Remember a time when you felt really good about yourself? How did you feel? Was your will to succeed higher when you felt good?

---

4. It's Simple: Change Your Lifestyle

While I was writing this book, my husband, who had no risk factors, had a heart attack, which resulted in a triple bypass surgery. I was plunged into the whole medical mine-field, and I knew all my theories in this book would be tested. This was evident when my husband and I met the cardiologist just hours after his heart attack. We waited nervously for several hours to meet the doctor and to get his assessment. When he finally arrived, his introduc-

---

8 Cromley, Jane. "Biggest Loser Explores Reality of Weight Loss," LA Times, November 13, 2006. www.courierpress.com/news/2006/nov/13/biggest-loser-explores-reality-of-weight-loss/.

tion to my husband was something like this; "Well, your life will never be the same. You'll have to change your lifestyle, your diet, be on drugs the rest of your life and, get yourself to a gym?" To which my husband replied, "We own a fitness center." The doctor recoiled and delivered his assessment in a matter of minutes and left. My husband's recovery was successful, which was bolstered by finding a different cardiologist, one who took the time to get to know his patient.

There are many lessons I could point out in this story, but the one I want to emphasize is a fundamental error of healthcare providers. With the best of intentions, doctors, nurses, and dieticians tell us to change our lifestyle and we'll be healthy. Using a behavior-change model, they'll try to determine how ready we are to change and then offer advice aligned with our readiness to change. Certainly no one knows more about the consequences of unhealthy choices than healthcare professionals, yet they too struggle to adopt healthy behaviors. With all their knowledge and daily contact with the consequences of lifestyle-based diseases, you would think health care providers would be "ready to change." So why don't they? That's a question I would have enjoyed asking our first cardiologist, who entered the hospital room with his belly first.

Change comes from within, as we learned from Dr. Maltz in the previous discussion. From this perspective, behavior change needs to be cultivated from within. You just can't flip a switch and have a new lifestyle. First, we need to focus on how we see ourselves, and second, we need to honor our childhood associations and the culture in which we live, which significantly influence our choices. We can't ignore them—they live within.

I fondly remember growing up in New York. My dad had died when I was six and my sister, who was eleven years older than me, was away at nursing school. It was just my mother and me. After church each Sunday, my mother and I would walk to the local bakery on 82nd Street in Jackson Heights and get the best New York crumb cake. We'd get back to the apartment and share those delicious morsels of sweet topping. It was a wonderful mother-daughter ritual. So, crumb cake will never be a forbidden food on my list. I cherish those memories and enjoy indulging in real New York crumb cake whenever I have the opportunity.

From my childhood I also learned to love egg on toast, pears and cottage cheese, lamb and lima beans, and asparagus and creamed tuna, all passed on to me from my mother. As I get older, I find I'm retreating to these foods more often. Maybe this is a phenomenon of aging. Regardless, my early childhood experiences are deeply rooted in my psyche. I know I can change this, but why deny myself the pleasure of pondering this wonderful mother-daughter ritual? This is good for my health.

Behavior change models fail to honor our upbringing and cultural biases; the focus is merely on the preferred behavior. Having lived in many parts of Canada and the United States, I can tell you there are plenty of different cultural influences. Canada's diet is influenced by the British and French cuisine with some Ukrainian influences in the central provinces. While living in Canada in my early adulthood, I grew to love cabbage rolls, French onion soup, Yorkshire pudding, Shepherd's pie, and butter tarts—foods I had rarely eaten growing up in New York.

As my career became more focused on health and fitness, my peers were all non-smokers, healthy diet gurus, and very active. I found it quite easy to pursue what is classified as a "healthy lifestyle," during this time. I lived in a metropolitan area surrounded by diverse recreational opportunities, hiking, swimming, boating, tai chi, and dance classes. Ice skating on the Ottawa canal was a peak experience. I urge everyone to experience this wonderful adventure.

When I moved to South Dakota, that all changed. I now live in a small, rural community with an agricultural-based economy. There's a lot of beef on the dinner table, the basis for the local economy. Many people live on or were raised on farms, so traditional farm cooking is the norm: meat, corn, mashed potatoes, gravy, and dessert. My husband, who was raised in a farming community in South Dakota, puts jam on every piece of bread he eats, even with spaghetti, something he has done since childhood. There are no dance studios, 24 hour fitness clubs, or climbing walls, but there is a lot of trap shooting, hunting, and fishing.

South Dakotans also reap the harvest by canning lots of fresh garden foods. Several summers ago, for the first time in my life, I picked corn, row by row with our best friends. We then shucked, blanched, and bagged the corn for freezing. We had such fun, and what a delightful taste in the middle of winter. This is all quite common in a farm-based community, but not New York City or Toronto.

The point I am trying to make is that our upbringing and culture molds deep personal preferences. These childhood experiences, I believe, will always be the foundation for one's diet and exercise patterns. The culture in which you currently live has a strong influence. We need to honor these experiences rather than demonize them. Even if you've changed some of your diet patterns, I believe you'll still have a tendency to revert back to your deep personal preferences—maybe modified but still preferred. Work from within those preferences and those of your current culture. This will breed more success.

Something to Think About

What food, eating styles, and exercise habits are linked to your upbringing and your community culture? How would you characterize your self-image? Does it make sense that lifestyle change would be more permanent if you felt better about yourself? What are the social-cultural influences in your current community? Does it influence your food choices and exercise patterns?

---

5. It's Mere Math: Calories In—Calories Out

The formula for weight loss, we are led to believe, is simple: Burn more calories than you take in. This, of course, is true, but it's never that simple. I remember in my twenties having a nearly "perfect" low-calorie, low-fat diet with the rare indulgence. I ran three miles four times a week and taught up to ten fitness classes each week. In those days my weight goal was 120 pounds, but I always hovered between 125 and 130 pounds, to my dismay. How could I eat so well, exercise so much, and not be 120? Plus, after even one small indulgence, I would gain a pound or two, or so it seemed. The simple math of calories in and calories out just didn't work for me, so I never confidently told my clients, "Burn more calories than you eat and you'll lose weight." A little part of me knew it wasn't the whole truth.

Now we know that hormones, metabolism, medications, and environmental chemicals often determine just how each calorie is treated in the body when it arrives. There are numerous individual differences that medical science just doesn't understand, some related to genetics, which determines at least 50% of our body shape. I always said to my clients, "We have as many differences inside our bodies as we do in our outward appearance." No two people will treat calories or nutrients exactly the same. You all know this to be true—you've watched how others eat gobs of "forbidden foods" and never gain a pound. These comparisons trigger lots of self-pity. "How come she can eat like that and I can't? It's not fair."

The real pitfall of counting calories, however, is the distorted relationship you create with food and exercise. Every morsel of food and exercise is assessed and calculated. You obsess and drive yourself and everyone around you crazy. It becomes the focus of your day as you agonize over each decision.

"I know it's bad for me but I'll just have a little bite."

"How many calories are in this muffin?"

"I have to walk an extra mile 'cause I ate a donut today."

As a fitness club owner, I was continually peppered with questions about calories and exercise. "Does this exercise burn more calories?" "How many more calories will I burn if I carry weights when I walk?" I witnessed one fitness club member traveling backwards on the elliptical machine. When I asked her why, she told me she'd read traveling backwards burned more calories. Do you enjoy going backwards? Is it natural for the body to move that way? These questions are more relevant than caloric expenditure. The truth is, the difference in caloric consumption is so negligible that it's not worth the effort and it's unnatural for the body—something you must respect.

Counting calories detaches you from the pleasure of good food and fun. In the March 2007 issue of *Health* magazine, the editor, Su Reid-St. John described why she loves inline skating. "When I need to clear my head or fill it with creative ideas, I put on my skates. Breathing deeply, I push, glide, push, glide—and suddenly I'm free from whatever was holding me back. My mind's open, my body's alive, and I'm filled with joy as I zoom along, soon drenched in sweat but loving every moment." The feeling she describes is what motivates her to skate, but the article was about ways to burn extra calories. The emphasis was on the eight calories per minute she burns, rather than the joy she experiences. The journalist missed the point.

Whether you're counting calories, fats, carbs, or points, it's destructive. The focus is in the wrong place. Stop counting the nonsense! Counting blessings is much more satisfying and will get you to a place where you feel good. Enjoy the pleasures of good food, friends, and a walk in nature's wonderland. Pleasure is a more reliable motivator, and you feel good.

Something to Think About

Is your reason for doing exercise to burn calories? If so, is it an effective motivator for you? Why or Why not? Think of at least one physical activity you do or would like to do that is fun and enjoyable. How do you feel when you think of that activity?

---

6. Fear: The Primary Motivator

The primary motivator of the current diet template is fear. I'm sure you've heard many statements like these:

"At this weight, you're at serious risk of diabetes."

"You need to get thirty pounds off, now 'cause you're headed for an early grave."

"You'd better get your cholesterol under control. You're a one step from a heart attack."

"You'll be fat all your life if you keep eating like that."

There is some evidence that fear may work in the short-term, but it rarely leads to lifelong change. I bet we all know someone with heart disease or lung cancer who never quit smoking. That is hard to imagine, but let me give you an example of such a person. I spoke with a dialysis patient who said he has no hope, and therefore no motivation to change. "Living is not worth it," he said. He's scolded and told he will die whenever he doesn't conform to the regimen required to manage kidney disease. Perhaps so much fear has been instilled in him and others like him that they've given up hope. Could it be that healthcare workers are robbing patients of any hope and scaring them to death?

I was recently in my favorite coffee shop where a local teacher ordered his coffee and sighed when I asked him how he was doing. "I'm doing okay, I guess. I just had a physical, and my usually mild mannered doctor scared me. He told me I'd better lose some weight because I'm tempting death. I've been depressed ever since." The teacher went on to tell me how he hates fruits and vegetables and exercise. "I'm a meat and potatoes type of guy. I hate all the diet stuff."

I launched into an explanation of why the diet template is flawed. Within just a few minutes he understood. I told him that avoiding disease was not the reason for living, and doing something he hates would not produce long-term results. I wanted to get this man in a better frame of mind, so I asked him to think of things he does well and things that make him happy. I reminded him, "You teach others, have a wonderful sense of humor, you laugh, enjoy your family, delight at the thought of your grandchildren, and you're a great teacher." His demeanor started to change. I advised him to wear a pedometer, knowing he is very mobile during the day. "You may surprise yourself just how much physical activity you already get in a day," I told him. "Build your exercise program around what you already do. Forget the gym if you hate it."

We discussed the many dimensions of health and how joy, not fear, is a better motivator. By the time he left, his usual cheery smile had returned. I don't think it remained; he had a follow-up appointment with his doctor and more than likely his fear returned. I learned later he went to Weight Watchers and lost forty pounds. He gained it back.

Research done by Barbara Fredrickson, from the University of North Carolina, suggests that negative emotions, such as fear, reduce our ability to see options. On the other hand, joy and hopefulness broaden our views and enhance impulse control and clear decision-making.[9] Stop being afraid of dying because you are fat! Life can be fun even with disease and even if you're fat. Let's use joy and hope as our motivator.

Something to Think About

Has your doctor ever used fear or threats to motivate you to change your behavior? How did it make you feel? Have you ever used fear to scare someone into being thin? Do you think it is an effective way to influence life-long change?

---

7. Critical Self-Analysis

The diet template asks dieters to analyze their behaviors when they binge or crash on the program. "What triggered your binging?" "What was your state of mind?" "How did you feel after you binged?" A common response is, "I'm an emotional eater." Do we really know this, or is this just a convenient explanation that then becomes a self-fulfilling prophecy? In other words, what we think becomes our reality; we believe it to be true. When we believe it to be true, we then act it out. "I'm so angry and emotional, I must eat." So, you eat. What if it's a lie? Maybe you're not an emotional eater, but you believe you are and behave as if it is true.

It's also very common to blame fatness on some old emotional issue. "What issues from your past are making you fat?" "Is it your relationship with your mother?" "Were you bullied at school?" "Was your father emotionally abusive?" "Were you the middle child?" "Who is the demon inside of you and where did it come

9 Friedrickson, Barbara. "Positive Emotions" Session presented at the Appreciative Inquiry Conference, Miami, FL. 2004.

from?" I've been in the health and fitness business for thirty years, and I've asked myself these questions over and over. I don't know why I tend to struggle with weight. Like everyone else, I have a past that contains both good and bad experiences, but I've never figured out what demon causes me to gain weight. If I can't figure it out am I destined to be fat?

I remember watching Dr. Phil's TV talk show when he first introduced his Weight Loss Challenge based on his book of the same name. Part of his program was to understand how your past contributes to your weight. "What is your fat covering up—abuse, rape, or an emotional trauma?" I was pleading with the TV, "Please Dr. Phil, how do I figure it out? Will I need years of therapy to find the answer?" My dad was alcoholic and died young, and my mother had insecurities about her lack of education and money. There is no doubt my parents' behavior had an effect on me, but what do I do about it?

After years of self-analysis, stacks of self-help books and some therapy, I finally strayed from the notion that I had to figure it out. The victim mentality was gripping me. I felt trapped as long as I was still deciphering my childhood, so I let it go. Instead, I pondered my childhood, forgave my parents, and thanked them for my good genes, my passions, my insights, and all the good things they did on my behalf, including the tickles, the laughter, and lots of hugs and kisses. Once I let go of the grip of the negative past and pondered the positive past, I was able to move towards my best life. I have a choice. Regardless of my childhood legacy, I can live the life I want. That is my intention.

I'm not minimizing the pain some of you may have experienced in childhood, and certainly not the horror of traumatic events like rape and abuse. These are painful human experiences that I am incapable of truly understanding. But for others whose past experiences are not as brutal, I will ask you, while negative past experiences do have relevance, do they have to dominate? If we're consumed in our negative experiences, it's hard to find space in our brains to register the positive experiences. Why focus on only the negative experiences and not the positive ones? Positive experiences also contribute to your development. Ponder and analyze those happy moments.

My mother could be quite judgmental, but she was also lots of fun. As a single parent with no high school diploma, my mother worked two waitress jobs so I could go to the best camp in the Catskills for two months each summer. I am so grateful. I cherish her gregarious personality and her pure joy of living. Recently, I placed pictures of my mother, who is deceased, around the house capturing her in some of her funniest, most joyful, moments. Now, I pause and delightfully ponder her enthusiasm for life, a trait she passed on to me. I feel happy and grateful I inherited her joy for living.

What are some of your happy memories? If you had lots of trauma in your home, you may not have experienced many happy moments, so think of a teacher, playmate, relative, minister, school bus driver, or any other adult who made you feel good about yourself. These thoughts, although they may be only a few, are seeds of positive growth. Give them a chance to grow.

To conclude my argument about emotional issues and weight, I will challenge a common notion. Are you ready? We are in the midst of an obesity epidemic, or so they tell us. If damaging childhood or other injurious experiences are the cause of our weight issues, we are then experiencing a mental health epidemic and not an obesity epidemic. Right? There is, of course, no evidence of such a mental health epidemic. So how can we blame obesity on negative past experiences?

I do believe there are emotional issues related to weight, but it's more likely related to repeated diet failures. Our self-esteem gets beaten up badly with so many failures. Think of children on a losing sports team. Their spirits are deflated, and they make excuses to avoid playing another game. The same is true of repeated diet failures—you feel lousy and deflated. Now, this negative state of mind could magnify deep emotional wounds, but these deep emotional wounds are not the causes of obesity—they're magnified by chronic dieting. Is this starting to make some sense?

I was gratified to read the opinions of Dr. Martin Seligman, in his book *Authentic Happiness*. Dr. Seligman, who is often referred to as the father of positive psychology, suggests the evidence is weak to support the theory that childhood experiences cause difficulty in adulthood. He states, "There is no justification in these [research] studies for blaming your adult depression, anxiety, bad marriage, drug use, sexual problems, unemployment, aggression against your children, alcoholism, or anger on what happened to you as a child."[10] He cautions his readers not to become prisoners of their past. Dr. Seligman is very well respected and his arguments are worth reading.

Since I began to study Dr. Seligman's work and the work of other researchers in positive psychology, I now focus more on the things that made my family life great. We had lots of singing, dancing, and tons of praise. I got to travel all over the country, and I even lived in Puerto Rico with my sister when I was ten. I had my own horse, lived on the beach, and had lots of good friends. My mother sent me to summer camp and professional dance school and surrounded me with family. I have wonderful moments to remember from my childhood. My childhood demons may still whisper in my ear, but they're in balance with lots of happy memories.

Analyzing the positive experiences of my childhood is a conscious choice. My periods of self-doubt may be rooted in my childhood, but the person I am—vibrant, creative, and full of enthusiasm for life—is also part of my roots. Why not use what was right in my life to get me going, instead of analyzing what was wrong with my life, which gets me down? Which question would you rather pursue?

I suggest you remember the things that fostered the wonderful person you are. Celebrate the wonderful traits and characteristics that make you unique. Cherish wonderful moments from your childhood even if they are only a few. Follow your natural strengths and abilities. You are an exceptional person with incredible talents. You are strong and have managed to overcome childhood demons to live a good life. This type of thought therapy fires you up. It builds self-esteem and your sense of self-worth.

So, when you think you have faltered on your weight and health goals, stop and analyze what you've done right. Each day, we all do something right. This type of thinking builds personal power so you can be the best version of yourself regardless of your body weight.

---

10 Seligman, Martin, E.P. 2002. Authentic Happiness. New York: Free Press.

> ## Something to Think About
>
> Everyone does something right each day. What is something you do right, consistently or periodically, that is good for your health? What are some of your best personal traits? What is one thing you are grateful for in your childhood?

The Diet Template Leads to Self-Loathing

The seven strategies I outlined are part of what formulates the diet template that leads us to the Chronic Dieters Fatigue Syndrome. Collectively they spawn a breeding ground for self-loathing. You try hard to follow the rules, but you fail. You obsess about calories and fat and never get it right. You hate going to the doctor because you'll get *the talk.* Your spouse, parents, children, and friends ask, "Should you be eating that?" You cringe and want to tell them to shut up.

How about the times you expect to lose weight after a *good* week and you don't? Or you promised to start your exercise program on Monday and you didn't? Or you're only allowed 1200 calories and you had 1300? How does that make you feel when you don't measure up—fat, depressed and a failure? When you feel bad, are you tempted to give up and binge?

With so much focus on your failures, the inner critic gains power and takes over as the master of your thoughts. The inner critic is not a great motivator for behavior change. How successful can you be when you feel so lousy?

The Alternative: Whole Weigh

What is the alternative? *Whole Weigh* offers you a radically different template—one that professes several wholesome principles to follow rather than rules and encourages you to integrate these principles into your daily life. Most of all, *Whole Weigh* builds your spirit, and celebrates the joy of living.

- Your focus is on being well, not thin.
- You have a vision rather than a goal weight.
- You analyze what you do right, not why you binge.
- You live by principles and not rules.

You are inspired to change because the focus is on the best of you, not the worst. Your inner critic is demoted, and though it will always fight to be the master, it now has serious competition in the form of positive emotions and thoughts. This is radical in the domain of diets, but it is exactly what we all need.

Chapter 3

Whole Weigh Template: Prescription for Success

"You don't need another diet, workout manual, or personal trainer. Go within, listen to your body, and treat it with all the dignity and love that your self-respect demands."

– Dr. Wayne Dyer

Adele Briton, a British singer who burst onto the American scene in 2009, is a confident twenty-year-old. She is extraordinarily talented, with a voice described as honey, and she is large, not only in life but in body. She was interviewed on the TV show, *Sunday Morning*, on CBS. The interviewer made reference to her weight and how she copes in a skinny business and still remains so confident. She answered, "If you are not comfortable in your own skin, you are doomed."[11] You, dear reader, must be comfortable in your own skin before you can truly reflect radiant health and happiness. Let me remind you, you are beautiful, handsome and awesome. It's from this perspective that I introduce to you the Principles of Whole Weigh.

The previous chapter presented the flaws of the traditional diet template. Now we'll consider a new template for weight loss, based on seven principles that acknowledge the inter-connections between our mind, body, spirit and the environment. The seven principles we'll investigate are:

1) Well-Being: Balance Is Best
2) Self-Love and Respect: You are the Best
3) Positive Psychology: Think the Best
4) Law of Attraction: Attract the Best
5) Intrinsic Motivation: Joy Is Best

---

11 Sunday Morning. "Adele." October 26, 2008. CBS News.

6) Close to Mother Nature: She Offers the Best
7) Trust Your Body: It Knows Best

All strategies for Whole Weigh spring from these seven principles. They release you from the rigid, obsessive way of living to a more harmonious, joyful life. These principles provide a strong foundation to begin a new relationship with your body, food, and yourself. Let's begin.

1. Well-Being: Balance Is Best

Well-being is a state of human existence that balances and integrates all the dimensions of the human experience: social, emotional, intellectual, spiritual, and physical. With so much emphasis on health and disease, our physical health dominates. Weight, cholesterol, triglycerides, blood pressure, and anything else that can be measured become the focus. When these health indicators emerge as more important than anything else, we lose our balance and ironically become less well. Positive emotions, social relationships, intellectual stimulation, and a keen sense of purpose and meaning in our lives are keys to our well-being.

What we need to do is release the fixation we have on our bodies, medical measurements, and the fear of illness, and instead tap into the fountain of well-being—our minds and souls—the true healers. This does not mean your medical measurements are not important; it means our other dimensions are equally important. Our body and health will benefit from a more integrated approach.

Look at the dimensions below and seek to honor each dimension, for they are the building blocks to being well.

- Socially, we need to connect to other humans.
- Emotionally, we must learn to like ourselves just the way we are.
- Intellectually, we need to wonder about humanity, nature, and our inner being.
- Spiritually, we need to relish a sense of purpose in our lives.
- Physically, we need to nourish and strengthen our bodies.

- Vocationally, we need to use our unique talents for personal fulfillment.
- Environmentally, we need to be caretakers of Mother Earth and Father Sky.

Cultivating and nourishing each of these dimensions brings vitality, joy, and meaning to our lives. The research provides concrete support of these claims. Here's a sample:

- Praying for someone who is suffering from an illness contributes to his/her healing.
- Positive, upbeat people have fewer colds.
- Satisfying relationships makes you feel good and less likely to get depressed.
- Doing volunteer work improves your good cholesterol level.
- Close friendships and families is the number one predictor for personal happiness.
- Those who keep gratitude journals sleep better and are more likely to exercise.

Has your doctor ever prescribed prayer or volunteering to lower your cholesterol?

The story of Roseto, Pennsylvania, a small Italian immigrant community, illustrates the relevance of well-being over traditional health indicators such as weight, smoking, blood pressure, and cholesterol. Researchers Stewart Wolf and J.G. Bruhn compared heart disease mortality rates among three Pennsylvania communities and discovered that the town of Roseto had 40% fewer heart attacks. They launched an intensive study to determine why. The citizens of Roseto smoked cigars, fried their food in lard, ate salami and hard cheese, and loved to drink their wine. They had the same levels of obesity and similar risk indicators as the other two communities. So why did Roseto's citizens have fewer heart attacks? The only significant difference the scientists could detect was strong family and social networks characteristic of immigrant Italian families: close, extended families, inter-generational relationships, and lots of family support. These human connections seemed to make them less susceptible to heart disease regardless of their diet, smoking, and exercise patterns.[12]

It is important to note that this study was conducted in the mid-1960s. Since that time, Roseto has been suburbanized and the social connections that once contributed to their health have dwindled. Their heart attack rate now matches the national average.

Healthy social relationships, spiritual pursuits, and personal happiness have significant effects on our physical health, but as I told your earlier, your doctor can't measure it or write you a prescription for a happy relationship. You must prescribe it for yourself: a healthy marriage, volunteering, prayer, laughter, and forgiveness. It's all good for your health.

Application to Whole Weigh

Whole Weigh uses the dimensions of well-being to broaden your attention beyond calories, weight, fat grams, and your body. The physical dimension alone should not define your sense of self-worth or how well you are. Whole Weigh brightens all the dimensions of wellness that flavor the essence of who you are.

With this is mind, your annual physical with your doctor is not adequate. It's an assessment of your body only. Whole Weigh provides a simple explanation and assessment tool so you can connect with your whole self. This will help you discover your true magnificence.

Something to Think About

Describe how you feel about your body. Does your body define your self-worth? What have you avoided because of your body size and/or shape? Do you emphasize your body more than the other dimensions of wellness?

---

12 Bruhn, John, G. and Wolf, Stewart. 2003. The Story of Roseto: An Anatomy of Health. Norman: University of Oklahoma Press.

2. Self-Love and Respect: You Are the Best

Dr. Maltz, who I referred to in the previous chapter, noted "you can never rise higher than your self-image."[13] A positive self-image is not easy to come by when you've had repeated diet failures. It leaves us feeling depressed, miserable, and hopeless. We fake our feelings, with smiles and laughter despite our internal misery. It's hard to feel good about yourself when you dislike your body, and your mind is preoccupied with thoughts that suggest, "I'm not good enough".

At this point, I want to clarify that there are subtle differences between self-image, self-esteem, self-love, self-respect and self-acceptance, but they're all interrelated. We need to love, accept and respect ourselves so our self-image and self-esteem are healthy and whole. Ultimately, when you feel good about yourself, doubt and fear are on simmer and you're more likely to feel confident about sharing your unique gifts and insights with the world. That's a good thing.

The focus of this discussion is self-love and respect. To be clear, self-love and respect are not the same as "putting yourself first" or "looking out for number one". This way of thinking generally comes from a feeling of sacrifice that over times breeds resentment and blame. "No one appreciates me." "We always do what you want." That type of thinking expresses a lack of self-love that we attempt to correct by moving to the front of the line. Putting yourself first because you resent being ignored or overlooked is not a virtue of self-love.

When you are in a state of mind of self-love and respect, you don't judge yourself as good or bad. You see yourself in a positive light regardless of your past history. You can forgive yourself and others for transgressions. You have a quiet confidence that doesn't need to boast or defend. You have no need to make comparisons between you and others. No one is better or worse than you. You're comfortable with who you are. You recognize your unique traits and personal strengths and are not afraid to express them. You have no need to be perfect because you appreciate who you are, as you are. You don't obsess about failing or looking fool-

---

13 Self Improvement OnLine. October, 2008. www.selfgrowth.com/experts/Maxwell_maltz.

ish. You may have moments of doubt but you are resilient and bounce back. With an abundance of self-love and respect you have no need to judge others; this is a special gift. You're forgiving and show gratitude for all things. You want to make a difference in the world, not by sacrificing your dreams but by living your dreams. It's a beautiful state of mind and one that needs nourishing to fully experience.

The journey to expand love of self generally grows incrementally, but can be accelerated by a major life event or accomplishment such as, fulfilling a lifelong dream or a near death experience. However it happens for you, there comes a moment when you're willing to know yourself better. That's when you begin to grow from within and more easily ward off self-doubt and limiting beliefs.

The first step for chronic dieters is to stop dieting. You can't hate your body, and engage in restrictive dieting practices and expect to foster self-love. It won't happen. Self-affirmations, gratitude practices and minimizing negative conversations of all types including self negative talk and gossip are ways to facilitate steps towards self-love.

Another way to foster self-love is to discover your natural strengths. This will give your inner champion something to build on. A natural strength is an innate ability, talent, skill or way of being. It comes easily to you. You may express your strength so effortlessly that you're unaware of its significance. Maybe you're an exceptional organizer, a great photographer, or calm under pressure. Maybe you're physically talented, can easily remember details, or have a flair for design. You feel in sync when your strengths are engaged. Years of diet failure may have dulled your connection to your natural strengths because you're so focused on your body and your failures.

Chapter Six will help you discover your personality traits that reveal your natural strengths. All you have to do is read the description of the four different personality groups and you will intuitively know which group reflects your true nature. Once you become aware, you'll be reenergized as your focus drifts from your body to your incredible natural strengths. This increased self-awareness triggers positive energy, and self-love and respect begin to bloom.

Once I understood my natural strengths and dominant traits, I immediately understood how they were reflected in my life. The way I shop, prepare meals, and exercise are all a reflection of my strengths and traits; so are my professional pursuits, hobbies and friendships. Knowing my strengths also revealed the source of my inner critic. Your inner critic targets your strengths. My inner critic would whisper, "You can't stay focused. You're too critical. You over analyze and can't make decisions. You're a daydreamer and a scatterbrain"—things I was often told by my teachers.

Let me tell you, dear readers, there is some serious damage to the inner critic when you begin to appreciate your true self. My constant stream of thoughts was not the sign of a scatterbrain; instead, it's an active volcano of innovative ideas. I'm not indecisive—I need to be well informed before making decisions. I'm not being critical, I'm being informative when I am pointing out the consequences of decisions or actions. From this perspective, I began to respect and better utilize my strengths, rather than be defensive and insecure. Knowing your natural strengths gives self-love a chance to grow.

How does all of this relate to my weight loss struggles? My personality type craves variety and freedom to do my own thing. I love research and enjoy scientific analysis, so I always evaluate and assess things with a critical eye. When I joined a weight loss group, I would constantly critique the program and leader. "This program is based on old science." "The materials are hard to read and make no sense." "The leader doesn't know what she's talking about." This constant critical evaluation weakened my motivation to stick to the plan. And by nature, I don't favor groups; I like doing my own thing. So, weight loss groups were not a good option for me, but I tried many times.

I also find it difficult to keep a daily journal, and nearly every weight loss program requires you to write down everything you eat. That of course translated into failure. I let myself believe that if I could journal, I would be a diet success. But I discovered, the requirements of the traditional diet regime were contrary to my personal strengths and personality type. I resist routine and am easily bored with mundane tasks. Despite my best intentions, I would rarely get one day down in the journal. This revelation relieved me of the criticism I would hurl at myself when I didn't complete a day in my diet journal. This doesn't mean I can't journal—I now understand it takes a bit more effort. Most important, I know it doesn't represent a major character flaw. I'm okay.

Discovering my strengths and personality traits freed me from punishing myself over previous diet failures. I learned I wasn't likely to follow a plan. I have my own theories about dieting and am more likely to devise my own plan. I know I easily get bored with routine exercise and prefer exercising alone. I'm a big-picture thinker and am more holistic in my thinking, so it is difficult to target a specific behavior when I view our minds, bodies, and souls woven together. I felt so much power when I got a better sense of myself. This points the way to love of self.

I don't want to mislead you, my deep personal awareness didn't happen overnight. It took time to deeply understand myself and connect with my strengths. And it took longer to deflect my inner critic. Today, I can say I'm more in tune with my strengths. My inner critic has lost its bite, and my inner champion gives me a boost more often. I am feeling good about myself. When you feel good about yourself, you are coming from a place of personal power. Writing this book is a real expression of my strengths and I feel strong and growing in self-love and self-respect.

When you are aware of your personal traits and natural strengths, you have a better idea of what you can do that is more in sync with your strengths and less reliant on your challenges. "Less resistance, more consistent," is my motto. Flow with your true nature and feel the synchronicity. As it flows, it grows.

Application to Whole Weigh

Getting to know your true self helps to relieve you of guilt over past diet failures. You're more in tune with your true nature and natural strengths. This boosts your personal power, and self-acceptance. From that place, self-love will grow. Love thyself—this is the source of lasting change.

> ## Something to Think About
>
> Intuitively, what do you believe are your personal strengths? What are you doing when you are at your best? Are you currently using your personal strengths in your life?

3. Positive Psychology: Think the Best

Thank heaven for the advent of positive psychology. This emerging field of study has triggered wonderful changes in the field and practice of psychology. Negative emotions like depression and anxiety have dominated the research, but now the study of positive emotions reveal the amazing benefits of happiness, gratitude, amusement, serenity, and love. This is a critically important balance within the field of psychology.

Here's a hint of what we know: "Happier people may live up to a decade longer than pessimistic people and are 50% less likely to become disabled. Happier people, furthermore, have better health habits, lower blood pressure, a decreased risk of heart disease, and stronger immune systems than less happy people."[14] As an added benefit, when you're under the influence of positive emotions, you have more impulse control and clarity in decision making according to Barbara Fredrickson, a pioneer researcher in positive psychology. Hmm, impulse control—now that's a good thing, don't you think?

Here are more of Barbara Fredrickson's key research findings.[15]

- Positive emotions allow us to become more flexible and less rigid.
- Feeling joyful creates the urge to play and be creative.
- Joy builds friendships that become the center of social support.
- Positive emotions can undo lingering negative emotions.
- When positive emotions are in ample supply, they spiral upward. They generate resiliency, optimism, and life satisfaction.

---

14 Authentic Happiness Website www.authentichappiness.org (Retrieved April 12, 2008).
15 Fredrickson, Barbara. "Positive Emotions" A session presented at the Appreciative Inquiry Conference Presentation. Miami, FL. 2004.

As we progress with this discussion, it's important to make a distinction between positive attitudes and positive emotions. Attitudes are deeply entrenched and take longer to change. Positive emotions, on the other hand, are easier to access and available with only a moment of deliberate intention. You can choose a more positive emotion when feeling bad, even if it is only an incremental step. If you are angry because you forgot to show up for an appointment, you can choose to forgive yourself, release those negative feelings, and feel good about something you did right that day. "Peace is just a thought away"[16] states Dr. Jill Bolte Taylor, author of the book, *My Stroke of Insight.* In an instant, you can choose to let go of negative emotions and allow yourself to feel better.

Let me describe a personal example. My friend Shelly and I made a video while we were on our debut Operation Beautiful mission. (You'll learn more about *Operation Beautiful* in Chapter 4) We were posting a "You Are Beautiful" message in the women's public washroom at our local Wal-Mart. Months later at the urging of Caitlin Boyle the founder of Operation Beautiful, I uploaded the video to YouTube, a video site on the internet. Caitlin didn't know, but that was my first video on YouTube and with that came some excitement and anticipation. Days passed and I was feeling a bit blue about life in general. I was struggling to lift my spirits and get on with the task of writing. Then in the bottom corner of my computer screen came an email announcement that someone had commented on my video. In an instant I felt excitement. I followed the link, read the fun comment, and out of courtesy watched one of MyKee's videos. My mood had already shifted with the email announcement, but now I was laughing hysterically while watching two guys, one dressed as a woman with rather large breasts, dance and bounce to Lady GaGa's "Bad Romance". Thank you, MyKee. In an instant my mood and emotions shifted. Humor is always a good choice for mood adjustments and there's plenty of that on YouTube.

So, you can change your emotions in an instant. I know, at times, you may be in a deep negative state of mind and it takes

16 Bolte, Jill, appeared on Oprah, November, October 21, 2008. Chicago: Harpo Productions.

effort, but you can do it. If you're in a bad mood and you flirt with a happier emotion, you'll feel better. Music, movies, and laughing babies on YouTube, can trigger a positive emotional shift—a happier mood is just a click away.

Barbara Fredrickson notes in her book, *Positivity,* that you can deliberately increase your positive emotions, and when you do your mind will change the way it sees and interprets daily events. Positivity will also invade the spaces in your mind where negativity breeds. Your inner champion has a bigger stage in your brain, and your self-worth prospers.

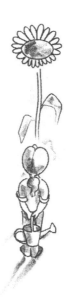

Positive Thoughts and Actions
Bring Positive Results

©Paul Liebau 1985
www.liebau.com

Application to Whole Weigh

Whole Weigh uses strategies that generate positive emotions. You analyze what you do right rather than reflect on your reasons for bingeing, and you keep a gratitude journal and not a food journal. You honor your personal strengths, and focus on things that make you feel good about yourself. What makes you so wonderful? What are your greatest attributes? What are you grateful for? These questions help to fertilize the brain so good thoughts prosper.

Something to Think About

Think of a time when you felt happy, relaxed, and optimistic. Describe your feelings and state of mind. How do you feel when you think of a time when you were happy? Do you think it's easier to change your behaviors when you feel good about yourself?

---

4. Law of Attraction: Attract the Best

"All that we are is the result of what we have thought." said Buddha. This is the premise of the Law of Attraction, which is a very simple concept—what you think about comes about. So what do you think about yourself most often? Is it mostly negative or positive?

As a chronic dieter, you likely have an abundance of negative thoughts about your abilities and your body.

"I hate my body. I'll never lose weight."

"I'm an emotional eater and my life is such a mess, I'll never get this weight off."

"I am so stupid, I never do anything right."

"I have no will power."

"I am such a bad cook, I have no imagination."

"I hate to exercise."

You think these thoughts over and over, and they expand and grow and become your truth. If you think you gain weight easily, it's true. If you believe you're an emotional eater, it's true. If you believe you're a bad cook, it's true. But with deliberate intention you can change those thoughts. Think good thoughts, and let them become your truth.

Here's an example of a deliberate intention to combat thoughts reflecting the notion that "I hate to cook."

> I enjoy cooking wonderful nutritious meals. I can easily follow a recipe and truly enjoy the results of my efforts. It is worth the energy when my family and friends tell me how wonderful the meal was. I feel good about cooking and preparing nutritious meals for my family.

These are the thoughts I peppered my brain with when I was challenged by my niece Laura. I always told myself I hated to cook. She challenged me to think differently and instead say, "I love cooking and I am good at it". With deliberate intention, I rewrote my script and told myself I liked cooking and was good at it, just as Laura suggested. The result is I am cooking more, eating out less, and experimenting with new foods and recipes all the time. People are asking me for my recipes, something that in the past never happened. I changed my thoughts and now enjoy preparing and serving meals.

"Energy goes where attention flows," states Michael Bernard Beckwith of the DVD *The Secret* fame. He says you need to, "… take your attention away from what you don't want, and all the emotional charge around it, and place the attention on what you wish to experience."[17] With that in mind, take your attention off your fat body and instead vividly imagine and feel the body you desire— healthy, light, and moving with ease. Let your thoughts take you in a new direction. In the meantime, love your body, just as it is. Feel grateful for the movement and the health it already provides. It has survived the punishment of yo-yo dieting and still allows you to breathe, move, and play. Be amazed by your body's resilience and the ability to heal.

This aligns your personal energy and emotions with your intention to be healthy, well, and fit. These positive thoughts about your health and body become a magnet for more positive thoughts and

---

17 Beckwith, Michael Bernard. 2006. The Secret, DVD, TS Production LLC.

guide you towards your preferred desires, a well, healthy, and fit body. This is how the Law of Attraction works.

Emotional Eating and the Law of Attraction

Now, consider the thought that you're an emotional eater. Is this really true, or do we accept it as truth because we've been told it's the reason we eat when we're not hungry? This statement seems to provide a reasonable explanation for such behaviors, but is it true? I always questioned the "emotional eater" theory, but could never adequately explain why. I just bristled when anyone would say, "I'm an emotional eater."

Recently, I perused my high school year book and had a revelation. My graduating class, from Evanston Township High School in 1966, was nearly 1,000 students. I looked for my friends and the longer I pondered the more I noticed very few of my class-mates were fat or even plump. I then carefully went through each page and identified possibly five people you might consider to be chubby—five people out of a thousand. If you believe the premise that being fat is caused by deep emotional issues and from emo-tional eating, then my graduating class had little or no emotional baggage. Do you believe that?

I don't believe we had any fewer emotional issues in 1966 than students today. We lived through the era of student protests, civil rights, the Vietnam War, and political assassinations. This was a time of serious unrest and social upheaval and a time when chil-dren had few avenues of escape from abuse. So, why would there be so few overweight people in my graduating class compared to today's graduating classes? Do you honestly believe that humans only became emotional eaters in the last thirty years?

As I mentioned in the previous chapter, if obesity is related to an emotional issue, then what we're facing is a mental health epidemic and not an obesity epidemic. NO! Our food sources, food production, food advertising, and lifestyles have significantly changed since 1966, not our mental health.

I said this before in the previous chapter, but it bears repeat-ing. If you have emotional issues related to your body weight, it's more likely associated with chronic dieting. Chronic dieting and repeated failures magnify our insecurities and make us feel bad about ourselves. We feel inadequate and hate our bodies. We are scorned in the media, school, and the workplace and bear the innuendos of our family and friends. This may lead to emotional eating, but I don't believe your weight problem started because you are an emotional eater.

The Law of Attraction contends, you attract what you think about. If you think you are an emotional eater, then you are. If you've given up and think you will always be fat, then you will. Why not give up this way of thinking? Instead, believe you are magnificent, with a healthy mind and body. You engage in wonderful nourishing habits that lead to good health and wellness. Start believing this, and it will become your truth.

"All that you are is a result of what you have thought," said Buddha. Be kind to yourself and think good thoughts about yourself, your body, and your health.

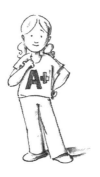

We Are
MAGNIFICENT.

©Paul Liebau 1988
www.liebau.com

Application to Whole Weigh

Whole Weigh helps you express your desires for a healthy, energized body. You'll create a vision of what you desire, and then be encouraged to generate thoughts and feelings in support of that vision. Imagine and feel what it's like to bounce up a flight of stairs, play with the kids, hike up the mountain, or paddle down the river with ease. Whole Weigh will encourage you to sense the joy of preparing and eating wholesome foods rich in nutrients and flavor. This is the Whole Weigh.

Something to Think About

Can you identify the thoughts you repeat in your head that diminish your ability to achieve your dreams? What do you think are the benefits of changing your thoughts to reflect more of what you desire and want in your life?

---

5. Intrinsic Motivation: Joy Is Best

Intrinsic motivation is that wonderful feeling you get when you're doing something that brings great joy and sense of accomplishment. You may hike twenty miles, restore an old car, finish a painting, or plan a fabulous party. You feel so good inside when you're done. Personal satisfaction is your reward; whereas, an extrinsic motivator offers a reward for demonstrating a preferred behavior. For dieters, the extrinsic reward is a lower number on the scale or a prize or recognition at a group meeting.

Extrinsic motivators are often used in schools to control behavior. Children will get stars or privileges if they behave. In the workplace, you'll get a bonus if you meet a sales goal, and at home children are promised a dollar for every A on the report card. Using rewards to motivate behavior seems like a sensible strategy, but research shows that extrinsic motivators inadvertently reduce intrinsic motivation—that wonderful sense of personal achievement without any expectation of a prize, money, or reward.

When we organized weight loss challenges at my fitness facility, weigh-ins were tough days for most people. Starving before and gorging after the weigh-in was the norm, and most people were disappointed with the results. Some people didn't lose weight because they had a bad week, and others had a great week but were disappointed when they only lost a pound. At the end of the competition, we'd reward people for losing the most pounds. Money and free gifts were given out during a celebration. Six months later, most people had regained their weight. We held these competitions repeatedly, and the results were always the same. So I learned what I already knew and what the research indicates; extrinsic motivators provide short-term results. I knew it deadened intrinsic motivation—people hated themselves and were embarrassed after losing weight and putting it back on. Some did this several times and eventually they stopped coming. The competition facilitated these failures.

In contrast, the first fitness program I developed in the 1970s was called "Fitness in the Park." We did basic fitness activities and once each week explored a new physical activity, such as hiking, dancing, swimming, and lawn bowling. My goal was to find an activity people might get hooked on. One member of the class, in her sixties, had been recently widowed and was quite depressed. She came to class with the intent of losing weight and getting fit. One Thursday, we were going bike riding. She hadn't been on a bike for years and was apprehensive. With gentle coaxing, I got her to join us. We loaned her a bike, and as a group we trekked out for miles. She loved it. Soon afterwards, she bought her own bike, and I saw her riding all around town. Within a year she took a bike tour in Ireland, where she met and married a wonderful man. That's what happens when intrinsic motivation drives you; it takes you places you may never have dreamed. Would the same story have happened if she were only looking for ways to burn calories to lose weight?

There is a substantial amount of research that documents the advantages of intrinsic motivation. In a year-long study, led by researcher Pedro Teixeria, Ph.D., of the University of Arizona, participants who experienced competency, interest, and enjoyment in physical activity had better maintenance of their weight loss regardless of the amount of weight lost during a four-month intensive weight loss intervention program.[18]

---

18 American College of Sports Medicine. Study Reveals How to Keep Weigh Off: Intrinsic motivation key to long-run success. News Release, January 31, 2006. www.acsm.org (Retrieved April 22, 2008).

Robison and Carrier, in their book *The Spirit and Science of Holistic Health,* explain the futility of extrinsic motivators such as rewards for losing weight. They explain that people need to find their joy—something that they love to do, that puts them in that state of flow. When in a state of flow, you don't need an external motivator. It comes from within.[19]

Avoid the lure of doing an activity because it burns more calories. Choose an activity because it brings you pleasure, gives you a sense of accomplishment, and gets you into your flow. You'll feel good, you'll have fun, and you're more likely to have long-term success.

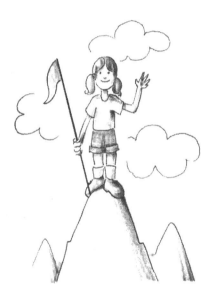

Reaching a goal is more rewarding when you've enjoyed the journey achieving it.

©Paul Liebau 1986
www.liebau.com

---

19 Robison, J., and Carrier, K. 2004. The Spirit and Science of Holistic Health. Indiana: Author House. p. 178.

Application to Whole Weigh

Whole Weigh recommends finding the *joy factor* in your choice of physical activity and food. That's your source of intrinsic motivation. And stay off the scale; it sabotages weight loss. It's an extrinsic motivator. Calculating pounds lost or gained, calories burned or consumed breeds controlled living. You're always struggling to live by the rules. Whole Weigh will tap into the wonderful feelings of fun and personal achievement. That is your fuel for change—the marvelous feeling you get when you do something that's fun. The scale will no longer determine your mood and sense of accomplishment. The benefit of intrinsic motivation is that it registers deeply within the brain and is often the primary ingredient for personal transformation.

Something to Think About

What are you thinking just before you step on a scale? Are you more likely to feel good or bad? Have you ever starved before a weigh-in and gorged afterwards? What do you think about that type of behavior—starving and gorging? Think of a fun activity or hobby you enjoy and finish this statement: I feel so good when I _____.

---

6. Close to Mother Nature: She Offers the Best

Mother Nature provides all we need to survive and thrive. She offers abundant nutrients in wonderful varieties and in the correct balance. She inspires us with glorious scenery, clear blue water, majestic mountains, and the sweet smell of pine trees. She beckons us to explore her wonder. She is beautiful and bountiful.

Mother Earth sustains life. We must trust Mother Nature, for we are one with her. The foods that grow upon her harbor nutrients to keep our bodies healthy. When scientists announce that blueberries are filled with antioxidants and good for your heart, it's hailed as an incredible discovery—but not to Mother Nature. When walnuts are discovered to be good for your skin, or celery good for circulation, it comes as no surprise to Mother Nature. She has offered all of these wonderful benefits in abundance from the beginning, for no profit.

Science is trying to figure out what Mother Nature already knows. So who should you trust: medical practitioners offering their best advice based on what they know at the time, or Mother Nature who holds all the answers?

Mother Nature is also our playground. Go outside and play. Lakes and rivers refresh our bodies and spirit. Drench yourself in the sensations of moving through water. Explore the majesty of the mountain and forests. Go out and walk upon the wonders of the earth. Stop and appreciate Mother Nature's art galleries filled with fields of flowers, grasses, and grains dancing in the wind. Ponder the sights and sounds of Nature's creatures. Bees gathering honey, robins tending to the nest, and buffalos roaming the prairie provide moments of awe and a reminder of the splendor of God's creations.

Application to Whole Weigh

Whole Weigh encourages you to eat fresh foods, preferably organic, without becoming a fanatic. When you're making choices, fresh is best, but frozen will do. Limit processed foods. Rather than routine exercise, go outside and play and enjoy the wonders of Mother Nature. Nothing is more exhilarating than riding the rapids, hiking in the woods, wading in a mountain brook or swimming in blue water. Mother Nature is always best.

Something to Think About

What do you think of the concept that Mother Nature knows best? Do you find it easy to trust Mother Nature, or is that a big step for you? Why or why not?

7. Trust Your Body: It Knows Best

The human body is an amazing complexity of interrelated systems that adapt remarkably well to challenge and change. Scientists try to unravel its mysteries. Although they grow closer with each passing day, they are still eons away from understanding all its functions and capabilities. We must then have an element of trust for the body because it knows more and knows best, just as Mother Nature does.

Trust requires a strong belief that our bodies are extraordinary and have the capacity to adapt, change, alter, and heal. Your thoughts need to honor and coddle the amazing feats of your body rather than be at war with it. As chronic dieters, we attempt to exert control over our bodies by depriving it of calories and punishing it with tons of exercise. If your starting point for weight loss is one of control over your body, then, as in any antagonistic relationship, it doesn't always go well. Harmonious relationships are more fruitful.

A harmonious relationship with your body requires appreciation for the health and pleasures that your body already provides. Our bodies are truly miraculous, and it is worth reminding ourselves of the gifts we experience each moment from our bodies. Below is how the voice of appreciation for our bodies might sound:

> My body can heal large and small wounds in days, adapt to cold and heat, and neutralize germs. It allows me to experience the smell of fresh air and the scents of nature that brings such pleasure. My sense of taste delights at the flavors of food and drink, and when I lovingly touch my spouse or child the sensations feel so warm and blissful. My body responds to the pulse of music, and I can dance to the rhythm with such joy. I can move my fingers across the keyboard to share my thoughts and write words with a pen that express my appreciation for my loved ones. I can balance on skis, run to the finish line, and laugh myself silly. My body alerts me of danger as a rush of adrenaline triggers an action. When I walk, my muscles so willingly move me towards my destination adapting to every condition, and when I breathe deeply I feel restored. When

I focus on my breath, I can feel a connection to a higher power that sends a wonderful sensation throughout my body that lightens my spirit. I can feel the pulse of my heart beating as it sends nutrients to each cell awaiting renewal, and each cell works collaboratively to ensure my well-being. I have an amazing body and I am so grateful.

Thoughts of praise for our bodies harmonize the body-mind relationship. Harmony reduces resistance, and the body-mind relationship flourishes. Without resistance, energy flows, and the body responds with good health and a wonderful sense of well-being. In contrast, when our minds continually complain and degrade our bodies, we create disharmony and resistance. That is not a good relationship, and we don't benefit.

Application to Whole Weigh

Whole Weigh encourages you to honor your wonderful body regardless of your weight, fat, cellulite, or disabilities. This is the best way to restore a harmonious relationship with your body. Next you must pay attention to the signals of hunger and fatigue as well as fullness, satisfaction, and energy. Be deliberate; ask your body questions. Are you hungry? Are you full? Do you need to move? The mind may convince you to have another bite, but your body will always be truthful: "I'd love to move right now." "No more food, I'm full." Get in sync with your body, for it can be trusted.

Something to Think About

What messages do you transmit to your body? When was the last time you complimented your body? Do you think there is some merit in thinking of your body in more positive terms? What would be the benefits of celebrating your body's wonderful qualities?

Summary
Standard Diet Template
Versus
Whole Weigh Template

Standard Diet Template	Whole Weigh Template
Weight loss is the primary goal	Well-being is the primary goal
Set a goal weight	Generate a vision of you at your best
Extrinsic motivators	Intrinsic motivators
State of mind: fear and self-loathing	State of mind: inspiration and joy
Guided by specific behavioral strategies	Guided by principles for living
Change your lifestyle	Integrate into your way of living
Do it to burn calories	Do it because it's fun
Follow the rules	Adopt the guidelines
Deprivation and restrained living	Appreciative and joyful living
Restrain and reduce	Explore and expand
Analyze negative behavior when you falter.	Analyze what you do right each day
Analyze your past for clues to weight problems	Appreciate the present moment and all it has to offer
Focus on physical dimension of self	Focus on multi-dimensions of self
Weigh to check results	Count your blessing for results

PART II

Whole Weigh Foundation

"Today is the first day of the rest of your life."

Whole Weigh is about to take you on a glorious journey—we're leaving now, as you read these words. You will experience new places and spaces. All your senses will be teased. The wonders of Mother Nature will excite you and make your journey more delightful.

We're traveling to a place you've dreamed of—a place where you no longer torture yourself about body size and weight; a place where you feel invigorated and strong; a place where your body feels alive and your mind is filled with happy thoughts.

You've longed for this destination for years. You thought about it, planned it, and even packed your bag with "stuff," only to find the baggage weighed you down. A few blocks from home, you'd turn back, saying, "I'll never stick to the plan. I hate my body. I'm destined to be fat." This is the journey of the chronic dieter.

On this new journey, you're required to leave the stuff behind. No baggage allowed! Free yourself from tortured and negative thoughts about your body and weight and all the reasons you're fat. Begin this journey from where you are right now. You will move forward in a hopeful state, encouraged and fully present in the moment. You will rejoice in this new day and new way.

Our sightseeing begins with a look at yourself and the characteristics that make you strong and unique. This will give your journey focus and help you travel light. You'll grow close to Mother Nature and savor her delights. You will walk, skip, or dance—whatever feels right. Then you'll think good thoughts about your life, your family and friends, and the beautiful world around you. You are on a journey to rejoice in your wonder, inspired by the pages of *Whole Weigh!*

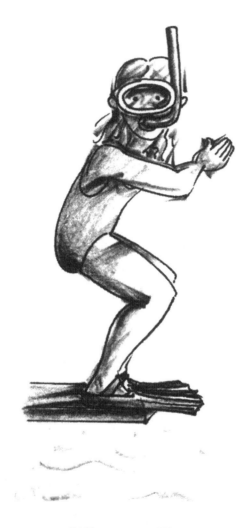

What are You waiting for?

Chapter 4

The Three Essential Practices to Quit Dieting

"You have to change the way you see yourself before you can change behavior."

– Bill Strickland

The quote above is the underlying premise of Whole Weigh; you need to feel good about yourself to change your behavior. When you feel good, you're more optimistic, content, and joyful—all resources for positive change. With this in mind, let's take that all-important first step and begin our journey with the three essential practices of Whole Weigh. Each of these practices is a beginning to change the way you see yourself.

Three Essential Practices

Chronic dieters have negative associations with food and their bodies. More than likely, a majority of daily thoughts have a diet theme. In order to begin to shift from a diet mentality to a more holistic approach one must shed three patterns spawned by chronic dieting. They are: diet-chatter, weighing, and negative body talk.

1. Stop Diet-Chatter

The traditional diet template keeps you thinking and talking about food, exercise, and weight. You measure, calculate, and record the quantity of your food. You constantly evaluate what's good and bad. You track the number of minutes of exercise and calories expended, giving preference to exercises labeled "fat burning." You try to control your behavior by analyzing bad moments when you indulge, binge, and stuff yourself. All of these behaviors generate incessant chatter in your brain and you spew it out in conversations.

"Oh, this has way too much fat."

"You can't eat that—it's loaded with carbs."

"Don't bring that into the house. I'll eat it."

"I look at food and gain weight."

"No birthday cake, I'm on a diet."

"I hate the stair-stepper, but it burns more fat."

This negative, debilitating practice ruins many a good meal and conversation, diminishing pleasure for you and everyone around you. It's boring and bad.

Diet chatter can also frustrate relationships and breed eating disorders. Your family is bound to tire of constant references to calories, fat, and body shape. Before you know it, you're scolding them for eating bad stuff, or they chastise you for going off the diet. You whine because you can't lose weight easily, but your spouse loses five pounds just thinking about dieting. This fosters lots of negative vibrations.

Children exposed to constant diet chatter learn from listening; fear fat, fear food, and constantly monitor and critique your behavior. As children age, dieting and body image consume their thoughts. Many fear weight gain and adopt a distorted body image, the seeds of eating disorders. These fears are being expressed in children as young as six. So please, STOP! No more diet chatter.

Diet chatter is a liability; it promotes a negative relationship with food, exercise, and your body—it's bad energy and it carries over into your relationships. So listen up—no more diet chatter.

2. Wean from Weighing

Weighing is a daily or weekly ritual for chronic dieters, and I know it's not going to be easy to convince you to stop weighing. We're conditioned to weigh often so our weight doesn't creep up. "How's that working for ya?"

Plenty of research tells us weighing often aids weight loss. But let me remind you, weight loss isn't the problem. Keeping the weight off is the main issue, and the ritual of weighing is a liability to weight maintenance. Why? Because numbers on the scale dictate our emotions, which are most often negative: anger, disappointment, depression, frustration, self-pity, and self-loathing. If you're a chronic dieter, then I know you rarely get on the scale and feel good. I am trying to convince you that feeling good is the best way to foster positive change. Weighing most often produces negative feelings. How does that help you?

Tracking your weight encourages you to focus on the wrong thing, the numbers on the scale. This external measure of your progress has the capacity to destroy your internal motivation. For example, after eating less and going for brisk walks all week, I'd expect to lose at least two pounds. If I get on the scale and only lose one pound, I'm disappointed. If I gain half a pound, I'm frustrated. If I lose four pounds, I rejoice—but subconsciously I know this is a green light for splurging. The splurge turns into a binge, and then I feel terrible. You have to eliminate the triggers that breed these types of thoughts.

If you participate in a weight loss program, I know exactly what you do on the day you weigh-in: you starve all day and binge all night. This is not a body-friendly ritual and does nothing to foster healthy habits. When you stop weighing, the feeling of success you get when you've had a good week stays with you. The good feelings grow—you're more optimistic, you laugh and play more, and you're motivated to make positive changes. A weigh-in risks all of these good feelings.

If we don't weigh, then how do you set a goal weight? You don't! A goal weight is just another trap. In my twenties and thirties, I was miserable at 125 because I wanted to be 120. At 130 pounds, I joined a weight loss program and meticulously recorded my food intake. I reached 124 and couldn't get below that number, despite being on a 1,000-calorie diet. The nurse looked over my food diary and scolded me for having more than one egg that week. Thirty years later, I vividly remember the scolding. I also remember getting mad, never returning, and feeling sorry for myself. Looking back, it's absurd to go through such misery and money over four pounds.

If I'd never stepped onto a scale, those four pounds wouldn't have mattered. I looked good and felt fit and healthy, but I let a few pounds dictate my emotions. I hated myself because I lacked the willpower to lose weight. I punished myself with more exercise, allowed the inner critic to bully me, and dressed to cover my fat. I focused on my goal weight instead of my well-being. Foolish!

Using numbers on a scale as the sole measure of your progress can lead to negative emotions that disable you. Change is almost impossible to achieve when you feel bad about yourself. You must wean yourself from weighing, and instead let your clothes give you feedback. If they're getting tighter, you're gaining weight—and that's all the feedback you need. One of my fitness center members Michelle said it best: "When you set a goal for yourself and you can't get there, you feel bad. You get discouraged. Just go with the flow. It will come off as it comes off, and you'll know when you get there." Michelle has lost over fifty pounds with that attitude.

Weaning ourselves from the scales can be challenging. Some people who've heard me speak on this topic totally reject the Whole Weigh philosophy because of this advice. I'll remind you, there is a 90% failure rate for dieting. Don't you think it's time to consider something radically different?

Stop weighing, and give up your goal weight. A vision of your ideal self will serve you much better than a goal weight. In Chapter 7 you will develop a vision of health and well-being. A vision moves you forward and inspires you with pictures in your mind of you at your best. Couple your vision with the analysis of what you do right each day and you have a whole new framework for health and well-being that doesn't require a goal weight. Here are just a few examples of positive analysis. (See Appendix I)

"I ate a sweet, juicy orange."

"I walked an extra mile."

"I played tag with my children."

This strategy generates positive emotions, and you begin to flourish. If you're tempted to step on the scale, all those positive emotions can turn to despair within one second. Positive emotions move you forward. Negative emotions suck you into a dark hole of the diet twilight zone.

I recommend going cold turkey, but more than likely you'll follow a gradual process, as I did. When we're conditioned to depend on weight as the sole determinant of progress, it's hard to imagine losing weight without using the scales. Nearly a year passed before I finally stopped weighing myself. A month or two would go by and I'd be curious about my weight, so I'd check. Each time I stepped on the scale I spent several days trying to shake the negative effects. The number wasn't always bad, but it shifted my focus from the joy of healthy living to the details of dieting. My thought process went like this: *I thought I'd be down a few more pounds. It's not fair when I work so hard. I might as well give up.* I always expected or wished for more, and inevitably I was disappointed.

This happened several times—and then one day I took my own advice and gave it up. I haven't weighed myself for nearly four years. I'm free of the mind games that accompany the ritual. In just a month or so, I went down a size in clothes, and in four years I've never gone up in size. I'm spared all the agony of weighing and still getting results. I can assure you, over time the number on the scale becomes less important, and you won't fret over a few pounds. This is great because a few pounds on the scale can trigger a binge, starvation, or another new diet on Monday, all driven by the measurement of weight.

With less focus on the scale and a goal weight, you're free to fill your brain with good thoughts about the things you do right each day. You're driven by a personal vision of you at your best, which you'll complete in Chapter 7. This gives you focus and excites you with positive emotions.

I hope I've convinced you. No more goal weights and no more weighing. Your well-being is what matters. This is assignment number two: Wean yourself from weighing.

3. Honor Your Body

The third essential step is to develop a loving relationship with your body. You've got to love it! At this moment you may be obese, overweight, or up a few pounds. Most likely, you hate your body. I'm telling you to love and accept yourself exactly as you are at this moment. Yes, I know you want to weigh less, but it won't happen with a negative relationship with your body. Hating your body serves no purpose and prevents you from being in harmony with your whole self, and this can add pounds. The emotions surrounding hate create negative energy that blocks positive changes in your life.

Take a few moments to appreciate your miraculous body—the temple of your soul, the tool for expressing moods and emotions. Think of the tingling you feel when someone you love touches you;

the butterflies you get when something exciting is about to happen; or the warning signals you receive when danger is present. Your body also translates the sweet smell of flowers, the sound of music, and the taste of chocolate. Your body has managed to survive crash diets, liquid diets, and cabbage-soup diets. You've starved it, stuffed it, and pushed it to the limit, and sometimes you did nothing at all, but your body adapted and supported you. These are all reasons to love it.

Once again, I won't pretend this is easy. Until recently, I hid my body under sweatshirts and baggy clothing. I never wore short sleeves or shorts. I always envied large people who went out jogging, dancing, or exercising and let it all hang out. I yearned to be that comfortable with my body. Why am I obsessing about hiding a size 14 body? I have a great, healthy body with curves. I needed freedom from those thoughts.

My attitude shifted in the summer of 2008, when my husband and I took a trip to the Sturgis Motorcycle Rally, one of the largest gatherings of motorcycle fans in the country, with lots of black leather and skin. I sat for hours and people-watched. I was writing this book, so took particular notice of big women in shorts and tube tops having fun. I wore blue jeans and an XL Harley T-shirt to cover as much of my body as possible. After several days of people watching, I final declared myself free of body shame. I bought a sleeveless top and wore it for the next few days, my flabby arms exposed. Over time it felt good. This was one small step for my body-acceptance therapy. I can't wait for my next Sturgis Rally: black, single strap T-shirt and tight jeans. Put my body out there and love it!

You have more potential to lose weight if you accept your body just as it is in this moment; it's beautiful and miraculous. Talk to your body right now. Thank it for enduring all these years and supporting your life. Listen to your body and let it respond to you. When you feel the urge to eat, pause and ask your body if it's truly hungry. It will answer. When you're debating about an exercise session, stop and ask your body, "What would you like to do?" It will tell you. It knows when you need to move. Listen to your body more and your head less.

Try this self-affirmation:

I love and accept myself exactly as I am. My body is beautiful and handsome. I am grateful for all my body does to keep me well. I love this body and can feel good health moving through it. Each cell is in sync with my vision to be healthy and fit.

My body relishes movement and moves with ease. It feels alive. I dress my body to express my joy in being who I am. I have nothing to hide. With each passing day I feel stronger and more vibrant. I am in awe of my body's amazing abilities to adapt, heal, and respond to my intentions.

I love my body, I love myself, and I feel good.

This type of affirmation brings harmony between your mind and your body. You need to have this type of relationship to release toxic thoughts, which produce stress, leach you of energy, and most likely cause you to hang onto the weight. Assignment number three: Love your body.

Operation Beautiful

The story of Caitlin Boyle captures the intent of the three strategies I just described. Caitlin started a movement which is reflected in the book she edited called *Operation Beautiful*. She captured stories of women who participated in her challenge to post anonymous complimentary notes in public places for other women to find.

Caitlin was fatigued from rigid dieting and the constant harassment of her own inner critic. She was challenged by her friend to cut-out the fat talk and she did. "After years of beating myself up, I couldn't believe that the answer to a happier life was so simple. All I needed to do was treat myself with kindness, love and acceptance."[20] From a place of self-love and acceptance Caitlin stopped fat talk and stopped weighing, and started loving her body and herself. She allowed her body to be its own master and now she eats intuitively.

---

20 Boyle, Caitlin. 2010. Operation Beautiful. Gothman Books: New York. P. p. 5.

Caitlin started a movement when she placed a post it-note saying, "You Are Beautiful", on the mirror in a public bathroom. She was feeling down and responded to an impulse to do something positive for herself and other women who might glance into the mirror. When she did it, she felt happy and as she describes, "giddy with excitement", hoping the next woman to read it would feel the same. She blogged about it and now it's an international movement called Operation Beautiful.

Caitlin challenges woman to place uplifting post-it notes in public places for other women to read, then photograph it and tell your story on her website, www.operationbeautiful.com. I posted "You Are Beautiful" notes in many public bathrooms on a road trip from South Dakota to Texas, and later to Chicago. Just like Caitlin, I was giddy with excitement. This is great therapy and a good way to implement the three essential practices of whole weigh. Start with a post-it note on your own bathroom mirror. You Are Beautiful. You Are Handsome. You are awesome. You are worthy.

Your recovery from chronic dieting starts with these three essential strategies. I urge you to practice them each day.

- Stop the Diet Chatter.
- Wean from Weighing.
- Love Your Body.

And don't forget to remind yourself... You Are Handsome. You Are Beautiful. You Are Cute. You Are Worthy and Well. You Have All You Need.

Chapter 5

Whole-Being: Balance Is Best

"The living self has but one purpose; to come into its own
fullness of being, as a tree comes into full blossom, or a bird
into spring beauty, or a tiger into luster."

– D.H. Lawrence

In this chapter I introduce to you "The Circle of Whole Being"
which illuminates a human being's wholeness. We are whole beings
who experience life through many dimensions; physical, social,
emotional, intellectual, spiritual, occupational, and environmental. Sadly, the physical dimension tends to consume our thoughts—
a hazard of chronic dieting. Yes, the physical health is an important dimension, but it shouldn't become the center of our human
experience. We "dumb down" our lives by obsessing over pounds
gained and lost, good and bad foods, fat burning exercises, and
cholesterol.

You must begin to connect with all the dimensions that make
you a whole person. This is an important step for recovery from
chronic dieting. Brighten your human experience by valuing positive human relationships, the wonder of nature, the satisfaction of
learning something new, and the glories of being one with a divine
source of goodness and love. Release yourself from the bondage
of the physical domain and rejoice in everything that makes you
whole. Allow your thoughts to dwell on beauty, love, gratitude and
joy. From this perspective you are in unity with your whole being,
from which the essence of life blooms. This is the *whole* in Whole
Weigh.

The following poem captures the sentiment expressed in the
above paragraph and throughout the whole book.

The Healthiest Couple*

They brush and they floss
With care every day,
But not before breakfast
Of berries and whey.

He jogs for his heart,
She bikes for her thighs;
They record their BP
For the lows and the highs.

He is loving and tender
And caring and kind,
Not one chauvinist thought
Is allowed in his mind.

They share household chores
And plan weekly for fun.
De-stressed and immunized
And screened from the sun.

They're home before midnight
Cause life is a ball,
Their diet? High fiber
And low cholesterol.

They avoid all cocktails
In favor of juice;
Cigarettes are shunned
As one would the noose;

They drive their car safely
With seatbelts in place
At home not one germ
Is allowed in the place.

They raise 1.2 children,
both sharing the job.
One is named Lila
The other is Robb.

And when at the age of
One hundred and three
They jog from this life
To one still more free,

As they pass through those portals
To claim their reward
St. Peter will stop them
JUST FOR A WORD!

"Stop here" he will say.
"You cannot go in.
This place is reserved
For those without sin."

"But we followed the rules,"
She'll say with a fright.
"We're healthy, near perfect
And incredibly bright."

"But that's it," will say St. Peter,
Drawing himself tall.
"You've missed the point of living
By thinking so small.

"Life is more than health habits.
Though useful they may be,
It is purpose and meaning,
Life's grand mystery.

"You've discovered one part
That makes humans whole
And mistaken that part for
The shape of your soul

"You're fitter than fiddles
And sound as a bell.
Self-righteous, intolerant
And boring as hell."[1]

---

[1] *Adapted from the Healthiest Couple by William Carlyon.
Source: Larry S. Chapman, President and CEO of Chapman Institute.

Whole-Being

Outlined below are the dimensions of whole being: the parts of yourself that make you whole. These dimensions are interwoven, not separate, and I only describe them separately so you'll see where and how to expand your focus to become a more whole being.

- Socially, we need meaningful connections to other humans.
- Emotionally, we strive to honor and respect ourselves the way we are.
- Intellectually, we wonder about humanity, nature, and our world.
- Physically, we covet good health and abundant energy.
- Vocationally, we use our unique talents for personal fulfillment.
- Environmentally, we are caretakers of Mother Earth and Father Sky.
- Spiritually, we sense a higher purpose and meaning for our lives.

Let's take a closer look at each dimension.

Socially, We Need Meaningful Connections to Other Humans

Humans are social beings who thrive on meaningful connections with other humans. These connections happen in various ways: a reassuring smile, a hug, an intimate conversation, a small gathering, or a community of people. Any shared experience with others, whether momentary or lifelong, becomes a human connection that carries meaning.

We learn about ourselves from these connections, even brief ones. A simple comment from a casual acquaintance can cause us to ponder and change our ways. Being part of a small group can reveal your true gifts. A disagreement with a close friend can provide moments of personal reflection. All connections, whether hurtful or joyful, are relevant and meaningful.

It's important to recognize that each of us has a unique way of expressing the social dimension. Some people enjoy a vibrant circle of friends, belong to groups, and love social gatherings. Others prefer one or two intimate friends and small gatherings. The human connection itself is important—not the number of connections. Those without meaningful connections are lonely and suffering.

According to research, people with strong social networks live longer and enjoy better health than people who are socially isolated. In fact, experts tell us our level of social connection is a good way to predict levels of health and independence as we grow older. Recall the story of Roseto, Pennsylvania, told in Chapter 3. Citizens in Roseto had fewer heart attacks because they had strong inter-generational relationships and large extended families.

Positive human connections help us to flourish and be our best. A sincere smile, a kind word, or a reassuring touch can change someone's day from despair to hope. It's to our benefit to generate positive connections; it feeds our spirit.

Replace thoughts of fat thighs, a big belly, and bad food with thoughts of cherished relationships, shared experiences, and friendly encounters with strangers. Infuse each of your human connections with kindness, joy, empathy, and compassion. You will be more whole.

Emotionally, We Strive to Honor and Respect Ourselves the Way We Are

Negative body images wreak havoc with our emotional dimension. How can you love yourself when you feel fat, dumpy, and ugly? Years of chronic dieting leave you with a legacy of failures, and your will to succeed is sapped. Fat and food consume your thoughts, and the inner critic becomes the dominant voice. Sadly we believe, "Once I'm thin, all will be well." I urge you to stop abusing yourself this way.

The divine truth is: we're all magnificent. Discovering this truth is part of life's journey. When we feel good about ourselves, our emotional dimension soars and life is good. To get there we need to be true to our natural strengths and characteristics.

"Nature never repeats herself, and the possibilities of one human soul will never be found in another," said Elizabeth Cady

Stanton, a pioneer for women's rights. We are all unique and see things in ways others do not. If we grow in confidence with this notion, our emotional dimension will flourish. Release to the world your incredible talents and insights, which are unique to you alone. Don't let fat diminish your magnificence.

I recommend reading *You Can Heal Your Life*, a superb book by Louise Hay, which will guide you toward self-love. Hay filled her book with delightful self-affirmations that make the soul tingle. She states: "When we really love ourselves, everything in our life works."[21] I learned that truth while writing this book. Fear and doubt about my ability to write, along with a plump body, stalled my writing. It took daily discussions with myself, my husband, and friends to combat this self-doubt. Eventually I triumphed by adding self-affirmations something I once believed was silly. I needed to appreciate myself and my unique perspective on wholeness, health, and weight. Self-affirmations helped me replace my messages of self-doubt with messages of self-worth.

Our emotional dimension flourishes when we begin to believe in ourselves and more easily deflect self-doubt. I suggest you begin by never denouncing, making fun of, or reinforcing stereotypes of yourself. You are not a dumb blonde, forgetful, or directionally challenged. You are not a bad cook, lazy, or too old. These are all things we configure in our minds. The more we recite them in our heads the more true they become. Recite, instead, your unique attributes: creative, caring, fun, adventurous, organized, thoughtful, responsible, loyal, etc.

Love yourself exactly as you are at this moment in time. When you do, your emotional dimension will flourish and your body will respond in kind because it doesn't have to carry the stress of fear and self-doubt.

Intellectually, We Wonder about Humanity, Nature, and Our World

The Arapaho say, "If we wonder, often the gift of knowledge will come." The word "intellectual" refers to wonder and curiosity, not

---

21 Hay, Louise L. 2008. You Can Heal Your Life. Carlsbad, CA: Hay House Inc. p. 9.

intelligence or formal education. We're born with a natural urge to wonder, seek, and learn. The curiosity of a young child leaves no doubt about our human desire to learn.

We accumulate information through our senses, and the brain filters and then stores information. We form perceptions and express them through our language and behavior. As long as one of our senses can extract information from the universe, we are learning. This is what makes the intellectual dimension so relevant to our wellness: we continue evolving and changing throughout our lifetime.

To be fully engaged in the intellectual dimension, you need to wonder, be open-minded, and willing to adapt your views. Humans, unfortunately, have a tendency to reject anything that contradicts a deeply held belief. If we wonder and seek new knowledge, we may discover many of our beliefs aren't true, especially those that limit our potential. "I'm too old." "I'm not good enough." "I can't walk that fast." "A belief is only a thought you continue to think,"[22] say Esther and Jerry Hicks in their book, *Money and the Law of Attraction*. We have the capacity to think new thoughts and grow and learn each day.

In this book, I'm asking you to accept a new way of thinking: don't weigh yourself, and don't set a goal weight. I suspect you still question the wisdom of my suggestion. That's a normal reaction, because shifting a mindset is a gradual process. But at least wonder and consider the idea with minimal resistance. This is the essence of the intellectual dimension.

Intellectual openness leads to high levels of awareness and understanding. We learn about ourselves, relationships, our world, and the universe. Formal education will aid this process, but so can your own curiosity. There are so many possibilities when your mind is curious, open, and full of wonder.

Further along in this book I will ask you to shed antiquated ideas about weight, weight loss, and health. I hope you'll be open to this beautiful oasis of new ideas.

---

22 Hicks, Esther, and Hicks, Jerry. 2008. Money and the Law of Attraction. Carlsbad, CA: Hay House Inc. p. 44.

Physically, We Covet Good Health and Abundant Energy

The human body, the expression of the physical dimension, is miraculous. Just for a moment consider our five senses, which allow us to experience the smell of lilacs, the sight of rainbows, the sound of a waterfall, the taste of a garden tomato, and the touch of a loved one. Each sensual experience is a gift from our bodies, every moment of the day.

Our bodies work to maintain homeostasis—keeping our cells balanced and working at their best. Our organs and glands orchestrate the ebb and flow of hormones, nutrients, and oxygen. Millions of cells receive life-sustaining substances from thousands of miles of blood vessels. Our bodies overcome disease, heal wounds and broken bones, and adapt to hot and cold. Our bodies facilitate the procreation of another human being. It's a miraculous feat. Pause and ponder the amazing capacity of the human body.

When out of balance, our body notifies us. We get signals when we're hungry, thirsty, in need of sleep, ready for sex, and when it's time to pee. If we truly listen, our bodies signal us when to move and what foods to eat and avoid.

During my entire adult life, my body has told me it doesn't tolerate coffee very well. If I have more than two cups, I get the jitters and a dizzy feeling in my head. But I love the taste of coffee and the ritual, so my mind ignores my body's warnings. Recently, after a thirty-year battle between my mind and body, I gave up coffee because it started to trigger heartburn. I could have taken an antacid to overcome the symptoms, but I would be ignoring my body's wisdom. That's never a good thing. There is a reason I get heartburn when I drink coffee. I don't know the answer, but my body does.

The human body is also wonderful at learning new motor skills. With practice we learn to walk, run, drive, skate, catch, throw, and ski. We learn to keyboard, skateboard, dance, sing, play a musical instrument, and swim. Our bodies are willing to learn any new skill we may consider and adapt to many grueling physical feats. It's only limited by our minds, which often suggests our bodies can't do it.

Beware of those limiting thoughts. "I'm too old." "I have bad knees." "I can't run." "I can't walk and chew gum at the same time."

NBC's *Biggest Loser* dispels many of those limiting beliefs. It's amazing what 300–400 pound people can do with their bodies—complete marathons, hike hills, climb, and balance for hours.

This point is illustrated by Gerry Hayes, the at-home winner from NBC's *The Biggest Loser*, season seven. Gerry and his wife were on the Biggest Loser campus for only two weeks. In those two weeks he learned the extraordinary capacity of his body despite being sixty-three and obese. He collapsed during an exercise session, but Bob and Gillian, the trainers on *The Biggest Loser*, still pushed him way beyond his perceived limits. With this lesson in hand, he went home and lost 177 pounds in six months and now runs 5K and 10K runs with his grandchildren. This is what he said during the show's finale: "Once I let my mind go and let my body do the job, it worked. My mind was holding me back." This reveals the interdependent relationship of mind and body. Make sure your thoughts expand your potential, not limit it. Your body is capable of so much more, including healing major illnesses. We must trust its wisdom.

Our bodies express all of the other dimensions of wholeness. If we're happy, sad, fearful, or content, our body interprets these emotions. If we're feeling angry or stressed about our work or family relationships, our bodies carry that stress, which often spawns illness. If we are not being true to ourselves, our body bears the scars. If we mistreat Mother Nature, our bodies ache. If we're awakened to our spiritual energy, our bodies will be filled with light and love. This is good for our well-being.

Be kind and true to yourself, and your body will glow with health and energy. Listen and trust the wisdom of your body, and your physical dimension will expand in the most natural way.

Vocationally, We Use Our Unique Talents for Personal Fulfillment

A vocation is the desire to follow the urge to do things that express your natural gifts. It can be described as a trait or a talent. It could be singing, cooking, organizing, leading, researching, sculpting, or designing. You may not be fully aware, but you keep doing these things because they feel right.

Looking back on my own life, I realize most of my jobs had three qualities: they were flexible, active, and educational. I was a waitress, camp counselor, fitness instructor, education coordinator, volunteer trainer, fundraiser, professor, and consultant. Each job included flexibility, movement, or travel, plus an element of teaching. I shunned jobs that required concentration, detail, and lots of paperwork. I took a course to be a real estate agent. Halfway through I knew this job was not for me—too much paper work, measurements, and calculations. I could have done the job, but I knew my strengths would be overshadowed by my distaste for paperwork and detail.

Doing what comes naturally is easy and spawns moments of true happiness, because you're "in sync." Too often we find ourselves in jobs thrust upon us by parents, counselors, or loved ones—work that goes against our natural instincts. Perhaps you're stuck in a job you hate because of health benefits, typical in the United States, or you live in small town and take what you can get. Whatever the reason, doing something foreign to your nature builds stress and resentment.

Your natural talents seek expression. They are generally the basis of lifelong dreams and personal passions. Here I am, finishing my first book at age sixty-two. I've longed to do this my whole life. Your natural urges rarely fade. They seek expression. Pull out your canvas and paint, learn to play the piano, join the community theatre, take a course, build a tree house, or go after the job you really want. Expand your vocational dimension by using your natural talents whether it be in your job, hobby, or volunteer work—it needs expression.

Environmentally, We Are Caretakers of Mother Earth and Father Sky

Every living thing on earth depends on Mother Earth and Father Sky. We can survive without parents, brothers and sisters, but we can't live without life-giving gifts from Mother Earth and Father Sky, says Eagle Man McGaa, the author of *Mother Earth Spirituality*. Mother Earth provides everything that nourishes our living cells, while Father Sky gives us air and rain. These life-giving parents work in collaboration with Brother Sun. They are to be honored and respected, just as we honor our parents.[23]

As you ponder this notion, you'll realize how the universe around us is interconnected. Everything on earth and in the heavens collectively sustains our ability to live. We must care for Mother Earth and Father Sky so we have the highest quality nutrients and air to nourish our bodies.

Nature is also a source of inspiration. Mountains, glaciers, waterfalls, and the ocean speak to us. The smell of a spring rain, the beauty of a rose petal, and the sun's warmth delight our human spirit. These moments of pure appreciation link us to Divine Energy. "Nature is the direct expression of the Divine imagination. It is the most intimate reflection of God's sense of beauty,"[24] says John O'Donohue, author of *Anam Cara: A Book of Celtic Wisdom.* Our spirits tingle with delight when we connect with the beauty and essence of nature.

This is why we must live in harmony with—and in honor of— Mother Earth and Father Sky. With each heartbeat, they nourish the gift of life. Gaze upon the beauty of nature every day and ponder the glory around you. This will heighten your connection to the Creator. Play upon the bosom of Mother Earth. Protect her and give thanks for the fruits she bears. Honor Father Sky, for he provides the air we breathe and the moisture to replenish Mother Earth. Let Brother Sun shine on your face and stream through your home. These things are life giving.

When you live to honor Mother Earth and Father Sky, you and all living creatures will flourish. This is our earthly connection to Divine Energy. Be in harmony with all God's creations, and your environmental dimension will expand.

Spiritually, We Sense a Higher Purpose and Meaning for Our Lives

Our spirits are naturally attuned to universal energy, most often referred to as God, Allah, the Great Spirit, or Divine Energy. Our spiritual dimension elevates our sense of purpose and adds signifi-

---

23 McGaa, Eagle Man, Ed. 1990. Mother Earth Spirituality. San Francisco: Harper Collins.
24 O'Donohue, John. 2004. Anam Ċara: A Book of Celtic Wisdom. New York: Harper Collins. p. 50.

cance to our lives. Each of us responds to this innate yearning in our own way and in our own time.

The spiritual dimension connects to all aspects of wellness: social, emotional, intellectual, physical, vocational, and environmental. Expansion in each of these dimensions enhances spiritual growth. This deepens our connection to Divine Energy and builds grace, which leads to love, inner peace, and "an awakening to your life's purpose," as described by Eckhart Tolle in his book, *A New Earth: Awakening to Your Life's Purpose.*[25] This inspiring book will quiet your mind and ego and elevate your consciousness, strengthening your connection to Divine Energy. I do recommend reading this book.

Chronic dieting promotes an obsession with the physical domain that hinders spiritual growth. Fixating on body image, calories, aging, wrinkles, aches, pains, and disease tilts the balance of wellness away from a full expression of our spiritual dimension. Our sense of purpose is blurred. Reread the poem at the beginning of this chapter—a reminder that perfect health habits are not the purpose of living.

To expand our spiritual dimension we need to generate positive energy—a channel to God. Judgment, resentment, self-doubt, anger, jealousy, gossip, criticism, and other negative states of mind deplete positive energy. Gratitude, forgiveness, love, acceptance, and peace generate positive energy and advance our spirituality. Positive emotional states of mind fertilize the soul and allow the goodness and love within us to expand. From this state of being, we grow in health and vitality.

The practice of mindfulness expands spirituality. For a long time I didn't understand this concept. I approached it artificially. I believed I was in the moment while playing, learning, and walking, but I wasn't truly mindful. Only when I read *The Power of Now* by Eckhart Tolle and participated in Oprah Winfrey's TV Webseminar with Tolle, did I finally get the point. I had to release my thoughts of moments in the future or past. The past is over, I can't do anything about it, and the future is yet to be, so no need to worry. All I have and know is now. I learned to quiet my mind,

---

25 Tolle, Eckhart. 2005. A New Earth: Awakening to Your Life's Purpose. New York: Plume.

sense my movements, and absorb the quality of the moment, even if I deem the moment to be stressful. These moments have value.

Daily meditation and prayer also expand our spiritual dimension; they align our spirits with God—the Divine Energy. These practices also promote healing, physical and emotional. Research has shown that with prayer and meditation, you can speed healing for yourself and others. You can relieve depression and grow in hope and optimism.

Although I promote these concepts, I'm still sporadic in my own practice. I am committed to generating positive energy through an expression of gratitude and appreciation and by practicing mindfulness. When conflict arises, I connect to the voice of love in my heart and coach myself, with the help of my spiritually attuned friends, to act from a place of love. The benefits are so worthwhile—peace and harmony, the voice of Divine Energy.

Spirituality grows like a child, with life experience as our lessons. Let this be the time you release the physical dimension's hold on you—a grip reinforced by issues with weight and disease. Choose to practice more positive emotional states and generate positive energy wherever you go; be true to yourself. Expanding your sense of wholeness will increase your self-worth, a healthier place to initiate positive change.

Suggestions for Becoming a Whole Being

- Think positive thoughts about yourself, your body, family, friends and foes.
- Speak only good words that lift the human spirit.
- Speak well of yourself and graciously accept compliments.
- Honor each human being you encounter. Like you, each is on a journey to find love, peace, and joy.
- Listen to your body; it knows best.
- Nourish your body with foods close to Mother Nature.
- Move in ways that make you feel happy.
- Be open to new ideas and the magic of the mind.
- Venture into nature and experience the wonder and beauty of all things.

- Honor and protect Mother Earth and Father Sky, who sustain all life.
- Be true to your natural talents and allow them bountiful expression.
- Dream, so your heart and soul have a voice.
- Experience the essence of each moment by being mindful.
- Be thankful for all things that make us whole and full of life.
- Pray and meditate to hear the voice of God.

Wholeness is a lifelong pursuit fueled by the soul's yearning for spiritual love and peace. Keep on the journey.

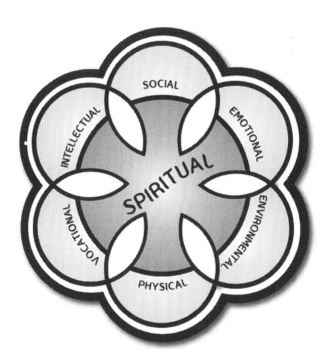

Something to Think About

Take a moment to reflect on your wholeness. Write one or two sentences that capture your expression of each dimension. Describe how you plan to develop in each dimension.

Socially what will you do (or already do) to make meaningful connections with other humans?	Physically, what will you do (or already do) to achieve good health and abundant energy?
Emotionally, what will you do (or already do) to honor and respect yourself just the way you are?	Vocationally, what will you do (or already do) to use your unique talents for personal fulfillment?
Intellectually, what will you do (or already do) to wonder and learn about humanity, nature, and our world?	Environmentally, what will you do (or already do) to care for Mother Earth and Father Sky?

Spiritually, what will you do (or already do) to achieve a higher purpose and meaning for your life?

Chapter 6

My Natural Strengths:
Be Your Best

"You already possess everything necessary to become great."
– Crow Indian Saying

Each of us is blessed with unique traits and special gifts that manifest through our hobbies, careers, leisure activities, and relationships. Some people love the excitement of riding dirt bikes, while others enjoy a solitary walk along the river. Some excel at the details of the family finances, and others fiddle with gadgets. Each scenario reveals clues to personal traits and strengths.

Another important step to recovery from chronic dieting is to recognize your natural strengths. Your diet failures have allowed your inner critic to dominate. To regain internal power and hear the voice of your inner champion you must connect to your natural strengths. Any intention you have to live your best life needs to honor your natural strengths for they are the source of your positive internal power. Determining your personality type will reveal your strengths.

In this chapter I describe the four primary personality types that have been documented throughout the ages. Hippocrates, Plato, Aristotle and Galen, from 450 BC to 190 AD, observed human behavior and independently described four similar groups that share common traits. In the 20th Century, Carl Jung, David Keirsey, and probably the most well known, Isabel Meyers and Katharine Briggs, observed, researched and confirmed similar observations, as those from ancient times. Over the years Meyers and Briggs developed an assessment tool called Meyers-Briggs Type Indicator (MBTI) that included sixteen different types. This tool has become the standard and is used throughout the world, most often in business and academic applications.

In 1950, David Keirsey correlated Meyers-Briggs to the four groups of the ancient times and developed his tool called Keirsey Temperament Sorter. He wrote the book *Please Understand Me* which popularized temperament and personality theory.

There are numerous personality and temperament assessment tools each rooted in the ancient philosophers, Jung, Meyers-Briggs and Keirsey. You can find assessments in books, workshops and online. Each assessment uses different words and symbols to describe the four categories: colors, shapes, animals, trees, birds, four directions and the four suits in cards. They are all very similar and worthwhile.

I chose the natural elements of earth, water, air and fire to represent the four personality groups, and I refer to them as My Natural Strengths. Each of these forces of nature has an energetic quality that reflects the energy of the corresponding personality type. I wanted to use natural elements to coincide with two main themes of the book—stay close to Mother Nature and be your natural self.

Read the descriptions and you'll recognize your most prevailing personality type. Once you do, you'll understand your strengths, motivations, personal preferences, and the source of many of your values. You'll also recognize the traits of others and know why you're different. This is a great revelation and just may reveal the nature of "personality conflicts".

I need to address one issue that often comes up when attempting to group people into categories. Categorizing can oversimplify the complexity of human nature. It can also influence people to exaggerate and/or adopt behaviors of the group they identify with the most. In addition, there's always the temptation of stereotyping people in each group. This happens all the time in school settings when we group children into ability groups—high performing and low performing. These concerns are valid.

There is always a danger of over simplifying, over identifying with a group, and stereotyping. It's all a matter of how you think. So listen-up; don't over simplify and don't over identify with one group. Use personality typing as one clue to understanding the complex nature of human behavior. Like snowflakes, there are no two people alike. Every human is unique, but like snowflakes we do have some similar characteristics.

The Strength Energies: Earth, Water, Fire and Air.

Read all four descriptions below and rank each element from the most like you to the least like you. There is a gauge at the end of each of the descriptions to determine your intensity of that strength energy. At the end of the chapter there is place to rank the intensity of all the descriptions and determine your profile.

When you read the descriptions be aware, you have traits of all four groups. You're merely attempting to rank the intensity of each group from high to low. All four groups are abundant in strengths, so one is not better than another. Just as in nature, earth, water, air and fire are dependent on each other to thrive. The same is true for you.

Most of you will easily identify the intensity of your highest and lowest energy groups. Some of you may be intense in two groups and have difficulty ranking them. That's okay. I am intense in both air and fire elements and sometimes it's hard to differentiate the two in my thinking and behaviors. Your second element will have an influence on your most intense element. It could soften or alter some tendencies in your primary element. So, you may read descriptions and not agree with all statements. That's okay.

One more warning, be careful not to choose a strength energy you would like to be rather than what you are. Be true to yourself and your natural energy.

***

MY NATURAL STRENGTHS

Earth Energy
Stable and Grounded

Those who reflect the energy of the earth are stable, grounded, realistic and practical. Like the earth, they're solid as a rock— dependable, loyal and trustworthy. Earth people provide structure and organization to counteract unpredictable situations. They're often the guardians of the family unit and may assume the same role in the workplace. Earth people tend to be literal rather than conceptual and more comfortable with the tried and true ways of doing things. Earth people are also patient and in no rush to change. It takes thousands of years to alter the earth and that's fine for those with earth energy. They like the earth beneath their feet because it's solid, secure and predictable.

Earth People are detail oriented, organized, and skilled at record keeping. Planning, preparing, and coordinating an event or family occasion is easy and enjoyable as long as they have advance notice. They cherish family celebrations and holidays, and are usually the chief organizer. They're the full expression of the saying, "a place for everything and everything in its place".

Earth people prefer predictable environments and routine tasks with clear outcomes. They are punctual, loyal, dependable, and responsible. They have a strong work ethic with a clear sense of right or wrong. They plan ahead, save money, and are usually, but not always neat and clean. At their job, school, or when volunteering, they like clear expectations and will frequently ask questions to ensure they're on the right track.

Earth people have high expectations of themselves and others. They will get frustrated and angry when others aren't meeting their standards, and may be described as critical. They may feel overwhelmed with obligations, worry about things that could go wrong, and may feel unappreciated because they're doing all the work.

Earth people are attracted to jobs in administration and management in the fields of business, education, health care, finance, banking, government, and law. Their desire for stability allows them to be content to work for one employer in their lifetime. They have a strong sense of civic duty and will often be associated with service clubs, church groups, or community groups that serve others. They follow the rules, respect authority, and seek stability.

You are likely earth energy if you... balance your checkbook, maintain the speed limit, arrive on time, hang-up your clothes, have a neat workspace, stick to the agenda, prefer routine, save money, make lists, plan a vacation with an itinerary, abide by the rules, honor deadlines, follow procedures, and generally do the right thing.

Natural Strengths of Earth People

Responsible	Family oriented
Consistent	Meticulous
Organized	Decisive
Adept at record keeping	In service to others
Attentive to detail	Guardians
Disciplined	Managerial
Industrious	Financially prudent
Advanced planners	Dependable and punctual
Producers of quality work	Diligent

Health and Wellness Profile of Earth People
Stick to It

Those with earth energy are more likely to follow the doctor's orders, read food labels, and faithfully schedule their annual check ups. In weight loss programs they are more likely to attend scheduled meetings and journal if it's suggested. They will follow instructions, recipes, and prepare shopping lists. When they are committed to exercise it becomes part of their daily routine, and they do it because it's the right thing to do and not necessarily because it's a fun thing to do. They'll look for exercise programs that are efficient and able to fit into their routine. They are keen on safety and will ensure everyone has their helmets on when riding bikes. They do best with a detailed plan of action that achieves a specific health goal, such as lower cholesterol, blood sugar, blood pressure, and weight. They are disciplined and like consistency, so they can more easily stick to a plan.

Earth people are more likely to prepare a balanced meal and sit down for family dinners. They will grow a garden, can and freeze the harvest, so they can eat right and save money. When earth people rally around a health and weight loss program they like to convince family members to join-in.

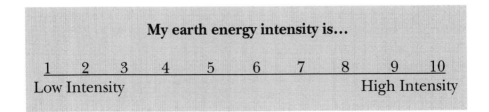

My earth energy intensity is...

1	2	3	4	5	6	7	8	9	10

Low Intensity   High Intensity

***

Water Energy
Nourishment and Relationships

Those that reflect the energy qualities of water are refreshing and nourishing. They make others feel good. Like water, they go with the flow, and enjoy the journey, where ever it takes them. Water people are compassionate, loving, and genuine caretakers. They're attuned to human needs and flourish in the service of others. They add a personal touch to all they do. Water people are imaginative and appreciative of all things that inspire, such as music, art, film, literature and nature. They may be avid gardeners and/or animal lovers. They notice and appreciate the beauty of nature.

Water people may be the super volunteer, always helping the underdog. They work in ways to foster the best in others, making great mentors. They are sentimental and cherish the small things in life that bring happiness. They are flexible, idealistic, and will always try to do their best. Water people cherish friends and family and seek to live a meaningful life. They will work to build consensus and will flourish in an atmosphere of cooperation.

Water people are sensitive and deeply connected to their emotions. The can be easily offended and overly concerned with what others may think of them. They are generous with compliments and in turn thrive when praised. They may find it hard to say no especially if it's for a good cause.

Their creative energy may lead them to a career in the arts— actor, director, author, musician, photographer, cake designer, chef, landscape designer, or painter. Teaching, nursing and counseling are other professions that tap into the strengths of water people. They can be very good in sales only when they believe in the product or service. Whatever the job, water people will deliver exceptional customer service. They care about people and will invest energy to make others happy and satisfied.

You are most likely water energy if you... are romantic, casual, artistic, like music and/or art, enjoy people and family gatherings, read fiction, watch movies, love nature, love animals, like to visit friends and family, take lots of pictures, collect things, easily remember details from the past, save things of sentimental value, stay connected to old friends, and converse easily with strangers.

Natural Strengths of Water People

Team Player	Optimistic and passionate
Compassionate	Sensitive to others' needs
Personable and friendly	Romantic and sentimental
Perceptive and insightful	Playful
Creative and artistic	Champions of the underdog
Nurturing	Respectful of nature and animals
Persuasive	Family oriented
Natural teachers and caretakers	Generous
Inspiring mentors	Effective Communicators

Health and Wellness Profile of Water People
Get into It

Water people are passionate about their health and optimistic about their success. They will seek support of others and benefit from group discussions that inspire them. They are more likely to journal about their feelings rather than food. They will invest a lot of energy in learning to understand themselves and their motivations. They will connect their physical health to holistic goals, for they sense the connection between the body, mind, and spirit. Physical activity has to be fun, flexible, and best when done with others. Water people enjoy the outdoors and nature, but can equally enjoy indoor activities especially in groups. Hiking, canoeing, yoga, pilates, tai chi, and activities with music and/or dance are appealing to many water people. Intense water people are open to alternative health remedies and mind-body practices.

They can be great cooks who are inclined to grow their own garden. They enjoy experimenting with new seasonings, flavors and recipes. Some may gravitate towards vegetarianism, motivated by animal rights and health. They have a flair for entertaining family and friends—sharing heart-warming food with music playing softly in the background, engaged in endless conversation. They are spiritually attuned always seeking to make a difference in the world.

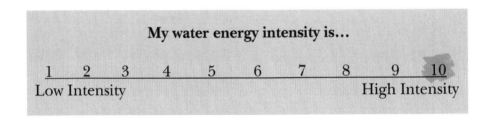

My water energy intensity is...

| 1 | 2 | 3 | 4 | 5 | 6 | 7 | 8 | 9 | 10 |

Low Intensity   High Intensity

***

Fire Energy
Action and Results

Those who have the fire energy have great enthusiasm for living. Like fire, they are energetic, spontaneous and intense. They respond to life's moments as they come. They are playful, courageous and full of adventure. They value independence, and need lots of variety and freedom to come and go. They easily organize a gathering or event on the spur-of-the moment. Because of this, fire people are great at crisis management.

Fire People are eager to solve problems. They thrive on the idea of resurrecting a project that's in jeopardy. When others give up, fire people turn on the heat. They have the skills to mobilize people and resources to make things happen. They can quickly adapt to evolving circumstances, making them very adaptable.

Fire people are intense and may appear impatient. They have strong convictions and can, at times, cause division among the ranks. Their love for adventure can sometimes become reckless and they can easily get bored with the mundane.

Fire people are energized by competition and risk-taking, and are often attracted to sports, speed, and jobs in the military, fire-fighting, police work, entertainment, construction or sales. Typically, they are not attracted to nine to five jobs. Fire people like hands-on work and prefer doing rather than talking about doing. Action and results are what matters to them. They spark others to take action, as well. They love surprising their family and friends and may be the entertainment at gatherings. Fire people are resourceful, natural trouble-shooters and always ready for action and fun.

You are most likely a fire energy if you... are energized, on the go, competitive, spontaneous, quick decision maker, can go from one activity to another with ease, challenge others, don't always pick up after yourself, enjoy parties, seek out adventure, stand out in a crowd, can easily entertain, laugh out loud, like roller coasters and things that go fast, do things well at the last minute, thrive on change, and for vacations prefer to head down the road and take it as it comes.

Natural Strengths of Fire People

Negotiator	Catalyst
Witty and humorous	Resourceful
Creative	Trouble-shooter
Entrepreneurial	Crisis manager
Entertainer	Motivator
Risk-taker	Versatile
Skillful	Adaptable
Results driven	Spontaneous
Energized	Enthusiastic

Health and Wellness Profile for Fire People
Wing It

Fire people enjoy anything that is adventurous, fun, and competitive. They like the outdoors but are equally comfortable indoors when it's related to a sport, competition, or anything that presents a new challenge. Their spirit of adventure will drive them to activities like mountain biking, hiking, camping, rock climbing, skiing, whitewater rafting, and scuba diving. They are energized if there is an element of risk. Competition is always a magnet and they will eagerly expend energy to beat a competitor. Most fire people are enthusiastic about physical activity, but will easily get bored with routine exercises unless preparing for competition.

They like foods that are simple and convenient and will try anything. "What the heck, you only live once." They will hunt and fish for their food, and will fire up the barbeque for some backyard fun and games. Their motive for good health is to keep active because their jobs and lifestyle depend on action and movement. At times they may be cavalier about their health, not because it isn't important, but because they believe you only live once. Life is meant to be lived; don't restrict your options. Fire people are intense about living life. They want to be free to enjoy what life offers.

My fire energy intensity is...

1	2	3	4	5	6	7	8	9	10

Low Intensity   High Intensity

***

Air Energy
Competency and Knowledge

Those who have the air energy are free thinkers. Like air, their minds are dynamic, and their thoughts are more abstract. They value knowledge and information, and love learning. As air is everywhere, so are the thoughts of air people. They love to think, gather information and generate new theories and models.

They may spend hours researching a topic just to satisfy their curiosity or to prove a point. They're visionary with interests in many areas. They're systematic thinkers, and can easily understand the interconnected relationships of all things. Air people are forever investigating, analyzing, and inventing new things or ways of thinking. They challenge the status quo, because there is always a better way. They're fascinated by technology, and they're either inventing or tinkering with the latest gadgets.

Air people strive for self-mastery which can lead to perfectionism. This can prevent them from moving forward as they search for the perfect solution. They're impatient with people who are resistant to change and will often have trouble communicating their ideas to others. They can become engrossed in their work or hobby and keep to themselves. Others may describe them as know-it-alls or aloof.

Air people are attracted to jobs that tap into their visionary thinking, such as inventors, scientists, planners, trainers, systems analysts, consultants, college professors, project managers, and journalists. They value autonomy and independence and therefore dislike being restricted by rules or procedures that make no sense.

Air people love interesting discussions and are bored by small talk. They can easily get lost in their thoughts and their work and forget to call home. They are loyal to their family, have a few choice friends, and need time alone to recharge.

You are likely air energy if you... enjoy debating ideas with others, collect information, love researching the purchase of a car, or appliance, read non-fiction, enjoy watching documentaries and news programs, have many ideas and unfinished projects, are a computer "geek" or "techie," or at least yearn for the latest gadget, like time alone, and love to share what you know.

Natural Strengths of Air People

Competent	Analytical
Innovative	Strategic thinker
Inventive	Conceptual
Curious	Principled
Rational	Visionary
Investigator	Intellectual
Logical	Objective
Flowing with ideas	Deep thinker
Knowledge driven	Ingenious

Health and Wellness Profile of Air People
Perfect It

Since air people are systematic thinkers, health and wellness is not separate but integrated into their whole being. Health is important, but it isn't always their first priority; knowledge and ideas always rank higher. They are constantly researching and critiquing new information to find the perfect approach to health and wellness. Because of this, they will generally devise their own approach to achieve health and wellness, foregoing the gym.

Most often air people prefer activities done alone or in small groups. They are more likely to be physically active when the activity fulfills another purpose, such as transportation to and from work. They enjoy activities or sports with others, but they really like those that require strategic thinking such as orienteering, geocaching, and martial arts. Air people are principled, so their diet and physical activity will be consistent with their firmly held beliefs. They may use technological gadgets to spur them on. But above all, their work, hobby, or research is the most fun of all.

They will forgo exercise and eating properly for days if they're consumed in their work.

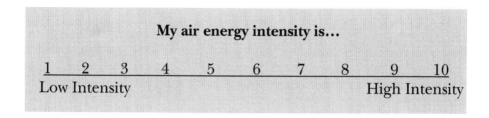

My air energy intensity is...

| 1 | 2 | 3 | 4 | 5 | 6 | 7 | 8 | 9 | 10 |

Low Intensity   High Intensity

***

What is your natural strength profile?

After reading the description of each energy group, determine which best represents you, remembering you have characteristics of each group. One or sometimes two of the strength energies are intense. Which element is the most intense? Which element is least like you. Record below and write this in your journal.

List all four strength energies in the order in which you think best represents you. Start with the most intense energy and finish with the least intense energy.

My Natural Strengths Profile

1._____

2._____

3._____

4._____

When you have chosen the order of the strength energies that best reflect you, reread the description and then choose the characteristics and strengths that you relate to the most.

My Natural Strengths

My most intense element is_____

My dominant characteristics and strengths are the following:

1._____

2._____

3._____

4._____

My second most intense element is_____

My second element adds these following characteristics and strengths:

1._____

2._____

3._____

4._____

My Natural Strengths Reflection

Considering your Natural Strengths, reflect on the following questions.

Self-Reflection

Write in your journal the following reflections: What do you aspire to do in your life? It could be dreams you remember from your childhood or a lifelong yearning. It could be an ideal job, hobby, or adventure. Maybe you are already doing it. Describe your dream and relate to your natural strengths.

Chapter 7

Imagine Me at My Best

"We must be prepared to act on our dreams just in case they do come true."

– Bill Strickland, Social Activist

Earlier in the book I asked you to abandon the idea of a goal weight; if you don't you'll remain trapped in the old diet paradigm. Perhaps you're asking, "How can I move forward without a goal weight?" The answer—generate a vision of your ideal self.

In *The 7 Habits of Highly Effective People,* leadership guru Stephen Covey describes Habit Number 2: "Begin with the end in mind." This is a simple premise that suggests you need to have a clear picture of where you intend to go: your destination. This is not a goal that you measure, it's a vision, a picture expressed through your senses and emotions. You imagine it and feel it.

A vision embodies your dreams, your wishes, and your ideals. It's filled with images of you at your best, doing what you love, and living your ideal life. When it's detailed and full of inspiring images, it serves as a magnet pulling you closer each day to your ideal self.

We are led to believe a specific measurable goal, like a goal weight, is the key to success, but is it really? Suppose you set a goal weight of 135 pounds. How are you going to get there? Are you going to skip meals, drink diet shakes, exercise compulsively, take laxatives, or down drugs? Will you consider surgery? Will you go on the South Beach or Belly Fat Diet or join Nutrisystem®? All these strategies will get you to your goal weight, but is it success? Is this you at your best? Is this what you dream for yourself? Stop and consider if 135 pounds is the goal or is the true goal to be well and healthy?

A subtle, but important distinction exists between setting a goal and developing a vision. A vision tells a story of you in the future—

it embodies your dreams and reflects your true self. It has life and radiates positive energy. A goal weight is stagnant and one-dimensional with no energy. It doesn't say anything about how you will get there, nor does it reflect your personal style. The scale determines your success or failure. If you don't hit your goal weight you've failed. You can't fail a vision. You become more aligned with it each day. Your vision is alive and calling you forward.

Vividly imagine and feel the energy of your vision using all your senses, and you will have success. Lynne McTaggart, in her book *The Intention Experiment*, states, "The evidence convinced me that we can improve our health, enhance the performance in every area of our lives, and possibly even affect the future by consciously using intention."[26] This requires a concentrated focus with a vivid picture of your ideal self, stated as if it were already true. You also need to sense your emotions that match your ideal self.

> "I am happy with my life, family and job. I have abundant energy, and a healthy body that moves with ease and thrives on nutrient-rich foods that I savor each day."

Using a vivid intention, vision, or visualization, whatever you want to call it, can reduce cravings, decrease blood pressure, ease pain, and improve performance. When your vision is clear with lots of positive images and emotions, you energize both mind and body to move in the direction of your intentions. This changes you in a way a goal weight can't. I want to make this clear, your vision is the centerpiece of your Whole Weigh journey.

Generating a Vision

This is a critical step. You may have glossed over other questions I suggested you think about, but don't skip this section. Your vision is the lightning rod for your new journey. You can't move forward without generating a clear, dynamic vision.

If you choose to ignore this step, don't expect anything to change. Here is my warning: you'll be trapped in the diet paradigm with a 90% failure rate. I urge you to commit yourself completely to this task.

---

26 McTaggart, Lynne. 2007. The Intention Experiment. New York: Free Press. p. 143.

It may be best to complete this task after you have finished reading the book, because there are many wonderful ideas in the following chapters that will release you from the traditional images of fit, thin, exercise, and diet. Your life is already mangled from these images and unrealistic expectations. Relate instead to images of glowing health, wholeness and beautiful bodies in all shapes and sizes. Do not be at war with your body. Be in harmony with your body.

In the previous chapters you learned how positive emotions, strong social relationships, prayer, and gratitude translate into positive physical and mental health. Therefore, when imagining you at your best, imagine positive feelings, relationships, and health, not weight. If you imagine good health, mentally, spiritually, and physically, your body weight will follow. You want to feel good about you and you want to be living your best life whatever your body size. You can still imagine less weight, but do it through the lens of glowing health. Be sensible, however, about your body image. Adjust your body image to what is healthy for you. Unrealistic weight goals keep you in the diet twilight zone, and this is not healthy. Release all of your previous weight goals, converse with your body, and listen. This may take some prayer and meditation, but you will be in harmony with your body, and that is beautiful.

I encourage you to read this section on generating a vision, then read the rest of the book and come back and complete your vision. Allow the images to form while reading the suggestions in the book.

You can generate a vision in one of two ways or do both.

1. Describe your vision in a written statement.

2. Create a vision board, a visual representation of your dreams for the future.

Choose the method you find most appealing—or use both. Whatever method you choose, do it with passion and enthusiasm, and complete this task within seven days. If you feel ready, do it right now!

Contemplate the following ideas for a vision statement or vision board with a few qualifiers. Please be kind to yourself and release any rules you are clinging to about dieting, food, and exercise.

Imagine You at Your Best

Close your eyes and imagine yourself at your best sometime in the future, several months or a year from now. Visualize what you're doing, tasting, smelling, and feeling.

- How do you spend a typical day?
- Ponder all the dimensions of wholeness, social, emotional, physical, intellectual, vocational, environmental, and spiritual.
- What are you doing that brings joy?
- How are you expressing your personal strengths?
- What are your accomplishments?
- How does your body feel?
- What positive emotions do you feel most often?
- If you were to paint a picture of you at your best, what images would you create?
- If you were to write a story about you at your best what would you say?
- What excites you most about your life in the future?

1. Describe Your Vision in a Written Statement

In your journal, handwrite your vision statement or perform this creative task on your computer in a fun font with added graphics. Make it special. Allow yourself at least thirty minutes for the writing process as you contemplate the questions I presented above. Release yourself of any rules you may have learned about vision statements. This vision statement needs to be descriptive, specific, and include your feelings and emotions. Use your senses as a source of inspiration. What do you see, smell, taste, hear, and feel?

Write your vision in the present tense, as if it's already true. It most likely will be several paragraphs long. When you finish, leave your vision statement where you can read it often. Daily is best. I printed mine on colored paper and had it laminated. See the sample at the end of this chapter.

2. Create a Vision Board for Your Vision

For your vision board, choose a sturdy surface large enough for your dreams, but small enough to move from room to room in your home or office. You want to see it every day. Mine is 14 x 14 inches. You don't have to be extraordinarily creative, just capture images that represent your ideal self. Find images on the Internet or in magazines that reflect your vision. I used images of hiking, camping, salads, fresh fruit, and vegetables. I added words to describe my feelings: joy, fun, passion, and success. I included a headline announcing my book is Number One on the New York Times Best Seller List and I'll be appearing on talk shows. Use the vision board to capture all the dreams about your health, your body, and your life—then keep it in front of you.

Whether you do a vision statement or a vision board, remember this will be your source of inspiration. Your words and images will help you move toward your dreams.

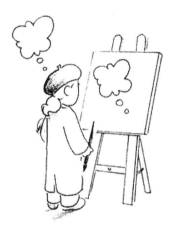

What you
Imagine
can come about.

READ IT—SEE IT—BELIEVE IT—BE IT

Here's how I described my vision:

> I am full of vitality and happy about the dawning of each new day. I am balanced in my wholeness, appreciating a quiet mind as well as a curious mind. My meditation brings me clarity and deepens my connection to Divine Energy. Most often my thoughts are positive, from a place of love for myself and others. I am generous with compliments and praise, and I express gratitude often. I have the courage to move beyond my fears, and I am doing the things I was meant to do, with confidence: writing, speaking, and teaching. My body feels strong and light. I have an abundance of energy. I eat foods that nourish my body in wonderful varieties. I never feel stuffed, and I experience no cravings. My urge to move my body happens easily and daily. Sometimes I walk vigorously, enjoying the outdoors in any weather, and other times I dance to music or practice tai chi. I enjoy hiking in the hills and running whenever I feel the urge. I find nature inspiring.
>
> I am gratified I'm able to use my abilities to inspire others. I appreciate the abundance of joy and financial security it brings to my life. My marriage to my husband is full of love, trust, and mutual support. My relationship with my adult children and step-children is very special and for this I am grateful. My life is wonderful.

Now that you have some ideas about vision statements, read through the rest of the book and come back to this. Remember, this is a critical step and signifies a new beginning. When you've completed your vision, go to www.wholeweigh.com and email me your vision.

PART III

Whole Weigh Principles

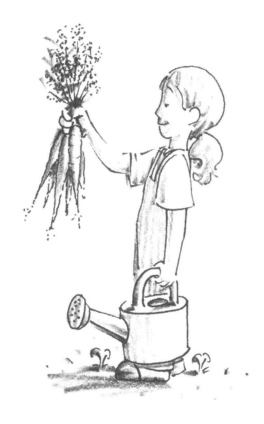

I Create What I Concentrate On

Chapter 8

Whole Weigh Eating

"Nothing would be more tiresome than eating and drinking if God had not made them a pleasure as well as a necessity."

— *Voltaire, French Philosopher 1700s*

Whole Weigh Eating is simple: eat close to Mother Nature, and enjoy the pleasures of food and the art of eating. We have strayed from simple wholesome nutrition because of our lifestyles, food processing, food advertising, and conflicting dietary recommendations. All of these factors collided in the mid 1980s to create health hazards that spawned the obesity epidemic.

Let's first examine dietary guidelines. You would think dietary guidelines from our government health agencies would be a sure thing, but they can be confusing, complex, and sometimes incorrect. You must be well aware of the changing rules—eggs were out, and now they're in; the same with avocadoes, nuts, and shell fish—they were out, and now they're in; and margarine was better than butter; now butter is better than margarine. The medical experts hate to admit their errors, and it's difficult to re-educate the general public when new research reveals those errors. You need to be aware that dietary guidelines are educated guesses about Mother Nature. It's worthwhile to remember that Mother Nature is the expert, not scientists.

In the 1990s, the United States Department of Agriculture's (USDA) food pyramid replaced the four food groups, and it has been a disaster. The pyramid encouraged a generation of people to get most of their daily calories from carbohydrates without qualifying the quality of nutrients and fiber. Six to eleven servings of white bread, pasta, rice, and cereals were recommended. What a big mistake. This was the same pyramid that demonized eggs, avocadoes, and nuts because of their fat content. The introduction of this food pyramid coincides with the increase in weight and diabetes in the United States. Check out the map on the Center for Disease Control website at www.cdc.gov/obesity/data/trends. You'll notice how the obesity rates jumped over a five year period following the introduction of the food pyramid in 1992.

Can you recall how your own dietary habits may have been influenced by the advice of the food pyramid? I do, because I ate lots of pizza, spaghetti, and bread, even though a little voice inside my head knew it was a lie. The guidelines gave you permission to eat up to eleven slices of white bread a day as part of a healthy diet. The 2010 USDA food pyramid recommends 6 ounces of grains with an emphasis on whole grains. Now, only three slices of white bread would be part of a healthy diet. The other three ounces would have to come from whole grains. That's quite a difference.

The US national school lunch programs were based on the 1992 guidelines, which allowed for an abundance of low-nutrient carbohydrates to be served. Pizza, spaghetti, chicken nuggets, French fries, hamburgers, buns, and deep-fried French toast dominated the menu. These foods are cheap and fall within the nutrition guidelines. Gratefully, the guidelines for US schools were changed in January 2011 to encourage more whole grains, fresh fruits, vegetables, and less salt and fat. But a whole generation will carry the effects of poor nutritional guidelines for years to come.

The second contributing factor to obesity is food additives. There are many that cause problems, but I will focus on high fructose corn syrup (HFCS), since it has received the most attention. High fructose corn syrup replaced simple sugar because of cost and convenience for the manufacturers. Then, HFCS began to show up in many processed foods because sweetened foods sell better. You unintentionally choose foods that are sweetened. You may not taste the sweet but you'll find you have a preference for sweeter foods. Food manufacturers are well aware of your preferences and lure you with sweetness. I believe our cravings are rooted in our overexposure to sweet tasting foods and low-nutrient carbohydrates. Check out the sugars in breads and see if the one you're currently eating is high in sugar compared to other breads.

In addition to sugars, the food manufacturers add substances that were never meant to be part of the food chain. They're added for preservation, taste, appearance, and cost reduction, not for nutrient value. Our bodies encounter these additives and get confused, and our livers get overworked. So we think we are "eating right", when we choose low-fat, high fiber processed foods, but we're duped. Consumers jointly share the blame with the food manufactures because we like convenience, but we pay the price with more calories, more cravings, and fewer nutrients.

The next major culprit is the food advertising industry. With extensive marketing research, these advertisers know how to position their products so we will buy more. They make us believe we must have sweet flavors in breakfast cereals and milk, not because sugar is good for us, but because sugar sells. Then, we're led to believe that drinking Mountain Dew is cool, and super sizing is a great deal for the money. Mother Nature does not have an advertising agency to sell nutrients.

The Federal Trade Commission calculates that children view 15 food advertisements a day, and 98% of these ads are for foods high in sugar and fat.[27] Research shows that viewers increase their preference for the advertised food. This, of course, is the intent of advertising and it works. How have you been influenced by food advertising? Do your children demand sugary cereals, dairy products and snacks?

The final factor that shifted us away from wholesome foods is our lifestyle. More women entered the workforce in the 1970s. With the added responsibilities, home cooked meals became less common in the American family. Fast foods, processed foods, drive thrus, and microwave ovens made busy lives manageable. It's hard not to take advantage of these conveniences when both parents work. However, all too often convenience dominates our food choices, not nutrients. The trend seems to be shifting back to home cooking. Hurrah!

These four factors mold our eating preferences. They are certainly not the only contributing factors to the rise in obesity, but they are definitely major influences. We need to stop basing our

---

27 Harris, L. Jennifer, Bargh, John A. & Brownell, Kelly, B. 2009. The Priming Effects of Television Food Advertising on Eating Behavior. Health Psychology. Vol.28, No 4 404-413.

food decisions on convenience, and sugary, salty tastes; instead we need to make food decisions based on nutrients. And above all, we must not let TV food advertisements dictate our food choices. Discover the flavor and convenience of Mother Nature's offerings.

1. Eat Close to Mother Nature

Eat close to Mother Nature. This simple guideline encourages you to eat foods close to their natural state. Eat fresh fruits and vegetables in season and meat from animals that feed in their natural habitat as often as possible. If you can afford it, go organic. If you're on a tight budget, buy organic foods you eat most often. I buy organic lettuce because I have a salad every day. Following this principle will make your cells happy, giving them lots of nutrients without asking them to decipher what's real and what isn't. Plus, your liver won't have to metabolize so much "junk."

Processed, non-nutrient foods are riddled with ingredients that play tricks on your cells and send mixed signals. For example, artificial sugars tease the cells with promises of sweet-tasting, simple carbohydrates for quick energy. The pancreas, responding to the tease, dumps insulin in your blood. The cells anticipate the arrival, but soon discover it was fake. Your cells get confused and begin to make mistakes. What do you do with a fake carbohydrate? Your cells don't know what to do, and the trouble begins. Remember it's not nice to fool Mother Nature.

Several other attempts to fool Mother Nature have backfired. Partially hydrogenated oils (Trans fats) concocted in a chemistry lab were once considered harmless when added to products like margarine to make them more solid. Then we discovered people who chose margarine to avoid heart disease were actually increasing their risk of heart disease. Altering the chemistry of foods is aggravating Mother Nature and you'll never win. Mother Nature knows best.

To evaluate whether prepared foods are close to Mother Nature, stop reading the labels and start checking ingredients. Labels are confusing and misleading. They don't reveal the quality of the food. You may choose a food with a low percentage of saturated fat according to the label, and not be aware of high percentages of sugars, toxic chemicals, and food preservatives.

Here's an example of how reading ingredients can help you choose foods close to Mother Nature. Keep in mind that ingredients on a label appear in a descending order from the most quantity to the least.

Kellogg's Apple Cinnamon Pop Tart Ingredients: Apple filling: corn syrup, dextrose, high fructose corn syrup, crackermeal, partially hydrogenated soybean oil, modified wheat starch, dried apples, malic acid, natural and artificial apple flavor, sugar, pectin soy lecithin. **Pastry:** enriched wheat flour, partially hydrogenated soybean oil, corn syrup, high fructose corn syrup, sugar, dextrose, salt, cinnamon, leavening (baking soda, sodium acid pyrophosphate, monocalcium phosphate), corn starch, niacinamide, reduce iron, vitamin A palmitate, pyridoxine, hydrochloride (vitamin B6), thiamin hydrochloride (Vitamin B1) and folic acid.) riboflavin (Vitamin B2.) **Relationship to Mother Nature**: **Distant Cousin**

Quaker Instant Oatmeal Maple & Brown Sugar Ingredients: Whole grain rolled oats, (with oat bran), sugar, (natural and artificial flavors), salt, calcium carbonate, guar gum, carmel color, niacinamide*, Vitamin A palmitate, reduced iron, pyridoxine hydrochloride,* riboflavin,* thiamin mononitrate,* folic acid.* (*One of the B vitamins.) **Relationship to Mother Nature: Second Cousin**

Old Fashioned Quaker Oats Ingredients: 100% Natural Whole Grain Rolled Oats. **Relationship with Mother Nature: A Child of Mother Nature**

Which breakfast item is best? This isn't rocket science. Old Fashioned Quaker Oats has one ingredient, and it's 100% whole grain oats. You probably get the point but wonder about convenience. Change your mindset, my friends: they're all convenient. Pop Tarts take two minutes in the toaster, instant oatmeal takes two minutes in the microwave, and Old Fashioned Oats take two minutes in the microwave or five minutes on the stove.

The real question is: What food provides the most nutrients and the least junk? You eat to nourish your body, not to stop hunger.

If you're a parent, which food best nourishes your child in the morning? Find where the word "apple" appears in the Pop Tart list. It's the seventh ingredient in the filling, after all the sweeteners and oils. The front panel for this product claims "made from real fruit," but, oh, such a tiny bit of fruit. Please eat an apple if you want real fruit.

Being close to Mother Nature is the underlying principle for all of Whole Weigh Eating. There is no other guideline more important than this one. Follow this guideline as often as you can without becoming a fanatic. Fanatics are stressed out, avoiding all foods that are bad. "I can't go to your mother's for dinner. She's serves junk." That attitude is bad for your health in so many ways. Calm down and enjoy good food as often as you can. Let's face it, with our current lifestyles, convenience is important, but you can still make choices that maintain the fundamental principle—eat close to Mother Nature.

Applying This Principle

- Right now go to your kitchen and find ten items that are close to Mother Nature. If you can't find ten, go to the store and stock your shelves with Mother Nature's food.
- Shop at a local farmer's market for fresh foods in season.
- Plant a small vegetable and herb garden. You can start with potted tomato plants and expand each year.
- Choose foods with short ingredient lists.
- Avoid foods that say "enriched" and have ingredients that are not in your kitchen cupboards, such as hydrogenated oils, high fructose corn syrup, and sodium benzoate.
- Avoid low-fat foods. They have been altered from their natural state and often have additional additives to add taste. It's not natural. Trust Mother Nature.
- Go back to "scratch" baking. Bake your own nutritious cookies, sweet breads, and pancakes with whole-wheat flours, oatmeal, nuts, cinnamon, flax seed, and wheat germ. Homemade pancakes eliminate all the additives and are so easy and delicious.

- Ignore all claims on the front of food boxes. This is a marketing ploy and doesn't truly represent the food's quality. Read the ingredient list.
- Avoid juice drinks that disguise themselves as a juice. Eat an orange or choose freshly squeezed orange juice not from concentrate. Check the ingredients and you'll know the difference.
- Avoid artificial sweeteners. Research has associated artificial sweeteners with increased weight, not weight loss. Diet soft drinks make you fat.
- Avoid anything that says artificial flavor, it's a stranger to Mother Nature and therefore risky. Remember, never let your body speak to strangers, you're body will be abducted.

2. Eat to Nourish Your Body

The food we eat provides energy and nutrients for every living cell in our bodies. That's why we eat: no other reason. Hunger signals the body's need for energy and nutrients. The more deficient in nutrients, the stronger the signals are from our cells. When your cells are nutrient-deficient, you'll get signals; for example, dry, itchy skin, twitching, cramps, fatigue, cravings, and brain fog.

One of my fitness club members experienced increasing fatigue over several weeks. One day she experienced spasms in her fingers and limbs while exercising. The symptoms subsided, and she went home without telling anyone of her episode. While at home alone, her spasms returned. Frightened, she struggled to dial the phone to call her friend for help. The emergency room staff suspected drug use, but after much investigation they concluded it was a lack of magnesium. She had been taking calcium supplements. Turns out too much calcium and Vitamin D can decrease the absorption of magnesium, a vital mineral for muscle contraction, relaxation, and oxygen production. Often a lack of magnesium is associated with fibromyalgia, so take note.

Your body needs nutrients in balance. Mother Nature knows this and provides a combination of nutrients in the correct proportions for maximum absorption and function. So, it's best to rely on fresh food, not supplements, for your nutrients, or you risk getting out of balance. Supplements are okay for therapeutic reasons, but shouldn't be relied on for general nutrition.

Breakfast Food

I have tended to be quite gentle with my advice throughout this book, but when it comes to children's breakfast, I can become a bit belligerent. A donut is not a breakfast food, neither is a Pop Tart, or a bowl of Frosted Flakes® or Froot Loops®. These foods are like a bowl of sugar sprinkled with enriched grains. Froot Loops give kids "a sweet and fruity start to the day" says Kellogg's. Sweet for sure, since sugar is the first ingredient in the list, and there is more partially hydrogenated oil than fruit flavors. Hydrogenated oils are linked to obesity and heart disease. Let's make this clear, there is no fruit in Froot Loops and therefore, not a nutrition-rich breakfast; but sadly, millions of children start their days with this bowl of sugar.

Your child is targeted by the food industry, which spends many millions of dollars influencing their food choices, and in turn the child influences you. Stop permitting corporate America to educate you and your child on appropriate food preferences. These breakfast foods are high in sugar and low in nutrients and are sure to cause things like brain fog, hunger pains, lightheadedness—all signs of insufficient nutrients. The body gives substantial feedback when it doesn't get the nutrients it needs. Sadly, when our children get to school and have these symptoms, they load up on what's available in the school cafeteria—cinnamon buns, breakfast pizza, deep fried French toast, and sugar flavored milk. That's lots of sugar and calories for a scant amount of nutrients.

We eat to nourish our bodies. That is your first obligation to your child. Be a good parent and send them to school fortified with quality nutrition so their brains and bodies can function at their best. They will still have their personal preferences, but be sure they're nutritionally dense and low in sugar. Tell your child they will run faster and think better when they eat nutrition-rich food. I taught my children to feel sorry for those who ate cheap sugar filled cereals and they believed me. You have more influence with your children than any advertiser. Use your power parents.

Nutrition Deficiencies

When you don't eat nutrition-rich foods, there are consequences. Here is a list of symptoms that are often related to a lack of vitamins and minerals: dry hair and skin, fatigue, insomnia, hair loss, dizziness, brittle nails, mental confusion, restlessness, weakness, rickets, dermatitis, numbness, bleeding gums, poor wound healing, constipation, muscle spasms, growth impairment, immune impairment, irritability, loss of sense of taste, night blindness, cramps, and easy bruising. This, of course, is only a partial list. I remind you of this so you will recognize the importance of quality nutrition.

The reason you eat is to nourish your body. Choose nutrient rich foods, so your body can have a clear mind, good health, and an abundance of energy.

Applying This Principle

- Before you reach for a snack, ask yourself this question: "Is this food I'm about to eat filled with nutrients to keep me well and healthy?"
- Use an affirmation to guide your food choices. "I am a nutrient eater. I feel good when I supply my body with life-giving nutrients to keep me well."
- Listen to your body. It offers many signals that indicate a need for nutrients. It also offers many warnings of foods to avoid. Trust the wisdom of your body.
- If your family expects dessert, experiment with desserts using fresh fruit that you can grill or bake.
- Add wheat germ, flax seeds, nuts, seeds, and raisins to any flour or meat mixture. It boosts nutrients.
- Sit for a moment, close your eyes, and ponder the magnificence of your body and each cell that contributes to your physical existence and well-being. Contemplate the messages the cells send to you. What do you need to hear? Listen.
- To ensure an abundance of quality nutrients, eat close to Mother Nature and eat a variety of colors of fruits and vegetables.
- If planning a conference or a morning meeting, avoid sweet rolls and donuts. Instead, provide fruit, cheese, and 100% whole-grain products.

3. Savor the Flavor

Since the 1970s, North Americans have embraced the convenience of fast food, boxed food, and drive-up windows. We wolf down our meals in a matter of minutes, often while driving. This cultural trademark, along with dietary chatter and calorie counting, leaves us detached from food and the process of eating. We rarely enjoy the pleasure of meal preparation, the taste of homemade meals, or the ritual of family gatherings. Seldom do we linger over delicious natural foods, while sipping wine and engaging in rich conversations, as the French and Europeans do daily. Our culture has relegated eating to an inconvenient necessity.

Savor the flavor is a simple reminder to reacquaint ourselves with the ritual of eating. See, smell, swish, savor, and swallow are the five "S"s that encourage you to engage your senses and make eating an experience instead of a chore. These simple steps will also upgrade your digestion, since each step assists the digestive process. Our tendency to wolf down our food hinders the digestive process. Slow down, aid digestion, and savor the food and the people with whom you share your meal.

1. **See**, ponder, and appreciate the food on your plate. A simple prayer of thanks will begin this step. The sight and contemplation of food is the first signal to the brain to expect nourishment; it begins the digestion process.

2. **Smell** your food and sense the pleasure and anticipation. Odor molecules pass over the taste buds as you breath in. This is the second signal telling your brain to begin the digestion process.

3. **Swish** the food in your mouth and chew. This breaks the food into smaller pieces, heightens the experience of your taste buds, and allows enzymes in your saliva to begin breaking down the food.

4. **Savor** the flavor. Appreciate the food's taste and texture. This heightens the experience of your taste buds. If you commit to savoring the flavor, you're less likely to eat food that tastes bad or is only adequate. You'll soon discover that foods close to Mother Nature are rich in flavor.

5. **Swallow** without the aid of a drink, and then pause. This will ensure you chew your food thoroughly. Your esophagus and

stomach will be grateful, and more nutrients will be leached from the food.

Applying This Principle

- Pay attention to presentation of your food on the plate. Make it look nice. This adds to the experience.
- Say grace before each meal, and then comment on the food before you. This adds to the ritual of eating and establishes a relationship with the food.
- Drink your beverage, preferably water, before the meal or at the end, but not during the meal. This eliminates the habit of washing down your food with liquids instead of chewing completely before swallowing.
- Frequent your local farmers market and make it a goal to taste as many vegetables as you can that are fresh from the garden. The flavor will amaze you.
- Only a half hour for lunch? Slow down relax and enjoy. Munch on your meal for the full thirty minutes. Savor each bite.
- Avoid all distractions. Be in the moment with your food and aware of the process of eating. Make eating an experience. Oh, what good habits you'll teach your children.

4. Eat a Little Bit Less, a Little Less Often

This notion is as simple as it gets—eat a little less. It's a great place to start if you're serious about your body's health. If you reduce your bite sizes and your portions sizes, you won't have to calculate a thing and you will avoid that over-stuffed feeling you may get at the end of a meal. Plus, you won't feel deprived, because you'll be eating your usual diet, remembering of course, you eat to nourish your body.

Portion sizes in the United States have significantly increased over the years, and we've learned to expect large servings in restaurants. Fast foods restaurants market the super-size, hoping to convince us we're getting a great deal for our money. Sure, but it isn't such a great deal for our girth and health. I want to change your mindset. We don't need a lot of food to sustain health. We are grossly overfed. Think small.

Although I don't personally recommend surgery for weight loss, I have several close friends who've undergone the lap band procedure. Four years after the application of the lap band, my friends thrive on small amounts of food. When we dine out they share a meal and still end up taking food home. Witnessing this, I realize how little food we actually require to sustain health. Change your mindset: eat like a bird. You'll have less belly aching, lower food costs—and most importantly, you'll enjoy better health.

Next, try eating a little less often. This suggestion is targeting mindless eating, those times we eat for no reason. The food is there, so you nibble; you walk through the kitchen and grab something; or you're preparing food and you snack. These are examples of mindless eating. I'm especially prone to mindless eating because I work at home. When you have one of those urges, overcome it by checking in with your body: "Do you need to eat this now?" Your body will talk to you. Listen. Just this simple question can interrupt the mindless response.

I challenged the members at my fitness facility to overcome the urge for mindless eating at least three times each day. This strategy is not restrictive; it just gives you a goal to manage your mindless urges. You still have permission to do some nibbling so it won't translate into a guilty feeding frenzy.

When you put it all together, eat a little less, a little less often— a very simple guideline.

Applying This Principle

- Abandon the clean plate club and get used to leaving several bits of food on your plate.
- Order small sizes instead of super-sizes from fast-food chains. You'll save money and calories.
- Use smaller plates. Research has shown this simple strategy reduces portion sizes and calorie consumption.
- Eat servings of meat no larger than the size of a deck of playing cards.
- Add this mantra to your thinking or add to your vision statement: "I eat little and light," or "I eat nutrition-dense foods in small amounts for good health."

5. Make Water Your Preferred Drink

Water is the best source of hydration, and it's calorie free. The only other fluid nature provides is breast milk. Everything else from nature that supplies hydration is part of a food substance— fruits and vegetables.

If we stick close to Mother Nature, then all we need for hydration is water, fruits, and vegetables. Everything else—including soft drinks, energy drinks, fruit drinks, and juices—is unnecessary. Corporations, which sell these drinks, market their products to you to plump up profits, while you plump up your waistline. We don't need them.

I have to single out soft drinks and energy drinks, because they have no nutritional value. Fruit and vegetable juices have some nutritional value, but juice drinks that sit next to the juices in the grocery cooler are frauds. Please know the difference between juice and juice drinks. Read the ingredient list, and you'll quickly learn the difference. Back to my point: fruit and vegetable juices are related to Mother Nature, fruit drinks barely know her, and soft drinks and energy drinks never heard of her. The latter were concocted in a laboratory. Most are loaded with caffeine. Why? To get you addicted. The manufacturers claim it's for taste. Oh, please! Caffeine is an addictive drug. What better way to ensure future profits then to have you addicted to their products?

If you drink soft drinks and go a day or two without it, you'll have withdrawal symptoms: headaches, irritability, and tiredness. Why are we giving this drug to our toddlers and children? They become addicted to caffeine, and without access to the drug through their soda consumption, they can suffer withdrawal symptoms. Your children will get irritable, get headaches and have trouble sleeping. Eliminate soft drinks from your child's diet and yours. And no more diet soft drinks. They make you fat.

So what about coffee and tea? Yes, they have caffeine, but they're close to Mother Nature. They're made from plant or bean substances, and caffeine is there naturally. This makes it close to Mother Nature. In addition, coffees and teas are most often seen as adult drinks and are not offered to children as often as carbonated drinks.

Make water your preferred drink. It doesn't have to be your only drink, just your preferred drink. Before I made the decision to give up pop six years ago, I drank two coffees, water, and the occasional pop. When I dined out, I usually had pop, because I wanted a treat. Once I decided to make water my preferred drink, I felt deprived when ordering water in a restaurant. Eventually I changed my mindset. Instead of feeling deprived, I decided to be proud and brag about my decision: "I only drink water." With that change in mindset the urge to drink a soft drink faded. So now, water and tea are my only drinks, with an occasional indulgence in fancy coffees.

To make water your preferred drink, change your mindset. Water is refreshing and compatible with all bodily functions. Water is a collaboration between Mother Earth and Father Sky. All living things flourish with water. It's what God intended and nature provides. Don't be lured by marketing campaigns that try to convince you otherwise. You also must beware of flavored water and green tea concoctions. Drink water, unadulterated with no added flavors—just refreshing, clean-tasting water. Be proud of your choice and brag about it.

By the way, once you stop drinking pop for a period of time, like an ex-smoker, you can't stand it. The taste and carbonation leaves a bad taste. I'm never tempted to go back to drinking pop. It tastes like poison to me.

Applying this Principle

- Use a water affirmation to change your mindset. "Water is a refreshing, cool drink that replenishes my cells, making all my bodily systems function with greater ease. The purer the water, the purer my health."
- Be fashionable and environmentally friendly by purchasing one of the latest reusable stainless steel water bottles. You'll save money if you ordinarily purchase bottled water. Avoid reusing plastic water bottles because of the threat of leaching toxins.
- Consider a water filter for your home. This might be a simple container with a carbon filter, a faucet-mounted filter, or the reverse osmosis water filter systems. They'll improve the taste

of your water, but beware they also filter out important minerals. Consider taking mineral supplements if you drink bottled and filtered water.

- Feel proud that you prefer water. It is a great statement of your commitment to your health. This mindset will make the transition easier. What you think about comes about.

6. A Touch of Color

A healthy diet is colorful: red, green, blue, purple, orange, yellow, and even white. Lots of color means varied nutrients. Each color is a clue to the source of nutrients: the darker the hue, the richer it is in nutrients. Eat them all in their most natural state, closest to Mother Nature. When you do this, you'll get maximum nutrients in the right balance with other nutrients.

Adding color to your meals is easy. It's best to consider this when preparing meals, but often when the meal is on the plate, I check for color and then add radishes, tomatoes, beets, carrots, grapes, pickles, watermelon—anything to create a dash of color. The morning I wrote this, I prepared scrambled eggs and toast for my husband—yellow and brown. I needed color, so I scoured the fridge and added sliced tomatoes and a few chunks of muskmelon sprinkled with blueberries. The plate was rich with color— so much fun to see and savor, plus I added extra nutrients.

A colorful diet means a great variety of vitamins, minerals, and other nutrients. You don't need to know or calculate anything, just eat lots of different colors of food. It's so easy. Choose dark colors often because they're power-packed with nutrients. Wouldn't this be a great way to plan school lunch programs? Lots of color.

Applying This Principle

- Shop in the produce section with color in mind. You'll buy things you may ordinarily forget, like sweet potatoes, beets, and yellow peppers.
- Establish a goal of having three colors on your plate. Add a few small fresh vegetables, such as radishes, beets, carrots, cherry tomatoes, or pickles to your meals. Sprinkle herbs on chicken, fish, beef, pork or beans.

- Make fruit part of every meal. Add a slice of apple, orange, watermelon, grapes, kiwi, mango or cherries to the plate. Anything for a splash of color.
- Grill fruit kabobs with many different colors for dessert. Yummy!
- Prepare a fresh fruit salad or a vegetable salad with color in mind. Let your imagination go wild.
- Bonus! As often as you can, bring fresh flowers into your home and add them to your dining table. Flowers make mealtimes special and add vibrant color to your home.

Chapter 9

Whole Weigh Moving

"We don't stop playing because we grow old; we grow old because we stop playing."

– George Bernard Shaw

Just for a moment, consider the word *exercise*. Does it conjure up images of stair-steppers, treadmills, sit-ups, push-ups, weights, and balls? Do you visualize regularly scheduled workouts at the gym? For some people, working out is a way of life, and they truly enjoy structured exercise. The rest of us—about 89%—go to the gym with the best of intentions, and then drop out after six to twelve weeks. Why? We drop out because we get bored, feel intimidated, or we find it hard to commit to a routine.

If you're a gym dropout like me, then you must reframe how you think about exercise. To begin your reframe, consider *active living*, a phrase coined in Canada during the 1990s to help broaden the concept of exercise. Active living is "a way of life that values and integrates physical activity into daily life." This idea comes from research showing that small bouts of light-to-moderate physical activity from recreational, occupational, or daily chores offers definite health benefits. The active living concept frames exercise in a more palatable way to more people. Going to a gym and doing calisthenics is not the only way to get health benefits from physical activity.

Now consider what physical activities you enjoy. When I taught the course History of Physical Education to college students, I always told them about Galen, a physician, philosopher, and author from the second century. Galen said,

Enjoyment is one of the most necessary factors in nearly everything that concerns the welfare of the body, and if exercise is distasteful and wearisome, its physical as well as its mental value is diminished. Exercise is best when it not only exercises the body, but is also

a source of joy. This will contribute to the health of the body, mental excellence, and strengthen the soul.[28]

Galen felt exercise should delight the soul and be true to our nature. Based on this premise, I encourage you to reframe your concept of exercise. Do physical activities that delight your soul. Who cares if your activity burns 30 or 300 calories an hour? So what if you burn fat instead of carbs? It doesn't matter if you exercise for 10 minutes or 100 minutes. What matters is the fact that you're moving and enjoying yourself.

As you think about exercise, remember your natural strengths from Chapter 6. Consider physical activities you can enjoy that reflect your nature. Do you like spending time by yourself or being with others? Do you enjoy competition or personal challenges? Do you prefer team sports or individual sports? Do you lean toward vigorous or gentle movements? Are you routine or flexible? Your answers to these questions offer clues to your nature and will help you think of physical activity in terms of your natural preferences. Check out the book *8 Colors of Fitness* by Susan Brue. It offers exceptional insights into your personal preferences for physical activity.

Traditional exercise can be a great choice for some, but not all. Different activities such as yoga, hiking, bird watching, kayaking, rock climbing, bowling, softball, dancing, and bocce ball are worthwhile pursuits. Any recreational activity that gets you out of the house and moving is worthwhile. When you move in ways that delight the soul, they become part of your life much easier. You'll find yourself eager to do them. This is more enduring.

Whole Weigh Moving encourages you to consider a wide realm of physical activity options. Exercise in a gym is a very efficient way of getting a good dose of physical activity, but it may not be your way. Consider movement in all forms—whether part of your daily chores, work, or recreation. Every movement counts.

1. Go Outside and Play

I've always loved the quote by Shaw, "We don't stop playing because we grow old; we grow old because we stop playing." Play

28   Van Dalen, Deobold, B. and Bennett, Bruce L. 1971. A World History of Physical Education. Englewood Cliffs, NJ: Prentice Hall. p. 77.

delights our spirits and lightens the burdens of life. As I sit and write this inside the Denver airport, I reflect on the amazing time I spent playing with my step-grandchildren, Brandon, Shelby, Trinity, Noah, Ethan, and Olivia. They're my best playmates. I had loads of summer fun. I swung on swings, slid down slides, bounced on trampolines, tubed behind a speedboat, drove go-carts, and played water monster. The most exciting event for me was sliding down a huge water slide at Wild Water West. I agonized for twenty minutes at the top of the slide, but when I finally took the plunge, it was exhilarating and I did it a second time. Brandon and Shelby, my coaches, gave me encouragement, and I appreciated their patience and enthusiasm. That triumph emboldened me to go tubing behind the speedboat.

The summer experience with my grandchildren reacquainted me with my own childhood, when I learned to play hard. I continued playing most of my life, but at some point lifestyle changes and age crept up on me. I started sitting out. The grandchildren helped me kick it up a notch, and I'm so grateful. I vow never again to let anything, especially age and body image, interfere with my ability to enjoy serious fun.

Play fuels the spirit and generates lots of positive energy. The fresh air from the great outdoors fills the lungs, and you feel great. Relationships blossom and fun is the dominant mood. The fatigue you feel after playing hard outdoors is genuine. Don't spoil your fun by counting calories—measure each activity based on pure joy.

Applying This Principle

- Play backyard games like badminton, bocce ball, beanbag toss, croquet, ladder ball, and dozens of other activities. Make backyard game time a family ritual.
- Play catch with your spouse or children. It will keep you limber.
- Get in the water and play. Do water parks, wave pools, tubing, and slides. Forget your age and fat; put on a swimsuit and play.
- Join a sports league for adults: slow pitch, softball, volleyball, bowling, old-timers hockey, lawn bowling, etc.
- Build a snow fort and start a snowball fight. Make angels in the snow.

- Play with the kids: hide and seek, tag, hopscotch, stoop ball, kick the can, and jump rope. They will love you for it.
- Climb a tree and build a tree house.
- Play on the playground equipment with your children or grandchildren. No sitting on the sidelines watching. The kids will love you big time.
- Play counting games while walking the neighborhood. Count garages, windows, street lamps, trees.
- Search the neighborhood for the biggest tree, the smallest and all the different types of trees.

2. Do Something Extraordinary

Do you ever wonder why people put themselves through grueling endurance activities like marathons, triathlons, or the breast cancer sixty-mile walk? They do it for the sense of personal satisfaction and achievement. I believe that each one of us, deep inside, yearns to do something extraordinary, whether it's a physical feat, writing a book, learning a new language, or walking across the country. An extraordinary accomplishment changes the way we see ourselves.

Tait Mckenzie, a Canadian born and educated medical doctor, sculptor, and physical education teacher, sculpted "The Joy of Effort" for the Swedish Olympic Games in 1912. This sculpture and others he created captured the exertion of physical effort and the joy of accomplishment. I've always been inspired by his work.

Physical exertion is a satisfying accomplishment—one that exemplifies the joy of effort. But in order to achieve this you must go beyond your perceived limits. You may think you could never walk twenty miles, cycle a hundred miles, or run at your age. You can. NBC's *Biggest Loser* participants, who started at 300 to 400 pounds, completed a marathon only six months after starting their weight loss journey. Amazing! And my friend Karin's aunt is getting ready to climb Mt. Kilimanjaro for the first time at age 69. Don't underestimate your potential.

Recently, *Sunday Morning* on CBS featured extraordinary walkers like Barbara Jo Kirshbaum, a seventy-year-old woman who enters three-day breast cancer fundraising walks. Starting at the age of sixty, she has walked more than 5,000 miles and raised over a million dollars. Do you think she is motivated by caloric consumption? Heck no! It's her deep commitment to the cause and her sense of accomplishment that gets her going. It's extraordinary.

My stepdaughter, Pam, along with cousins and friends, finished her first three-day cancer walk in 2008. When I spoke to her, hours after she crossed the finish line, she told me she was tired, had heat rash, road rash, and her feet ached, but she felt extraordinarily proud of her accomplishment. She considers this feat, despite all the physical and mental agony, a highlight of her life.

Then there's the fourth-grade class at Filer Elementary School in Idaho. Each year they complete The Big Walk: fifty miles in five consecutive days. Physical education teacher Vickie Leach proposed this idea to her school board in 1992. As you can imagine, people doubted fourth graders could do the walk. In 2010, they embarked on their nineteenth year of walking. Many students who graduate from high school in that district recall The Big Walk in fourth grade as their most memorable school experience. Imagine how they felt crossing the finish line on the fifth day of walking. That's a major achievement.

I interviewed Vicki Leach for one of my physical education classes, and she emphasized one thing: "Push your students to do something extraordinary." Then she told stories of how children changed the way they perceived themselves. Some children or their parents had doubts they could finish. They crossed the finish line with aching feet, blisters, sore muscles—and a sense of exhilaration and self-worth money couldn't buy. The walk heightened their self-image. Parents, grandparents, and community members who once protested the notion that fourth graders could walk fifty miles now join the fun. There's joy in effort.

When you accomplish something that requires a great deal of effort, the rewards go deep; you are intrinsically motivated and your inner power oozes with confidence. Your sense of accomplishment is the reward, not the loss of 10 pounds—although that may happen, it's not what resonates within your soul. When you cross the finish line after a grueling effort, I am certain you're not celebrating the loss of 10 pounds, you're celebrating the accomplishment. So, do something extraordinary. Experience the joy of effort and relish in your accomplishment. This will change the way you see yourself.

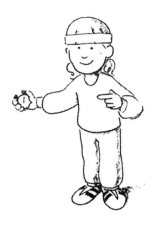

You'll never <u>really</u> believe in yourself
until you put yourself to the test.

Applying This Principle

- Register and train for a challenging, walk, run, bike, and/or swim.
- Plan a daylong hike with family and friends.
- Regardless of your age, run a block, then two, then three, then a mile. Keep running, like sixty-three-year-old Gerry Hayes from the *Biggest Loser* and seventy-year-old Jo Kirshbaum.
- Double your time on a cardio machine at your next workout.
- Walk fifty miles in one week like the fourth graders from Idaho.
- Hint: Get compression shorts made from spandex and Lycra. They make you feel like an athlete and research indicates they actually improve performance.

3. Move a Little Bit More, a Little More Often

ParticipACTION, a quasi-governmental agency in Canada, was established to promote physical activity to Canadians. They coined the phrase "move a little bit more, a little more often" to promote active living, an integrated approach to including physical activity in your daily life. You can lower your cholesterol, decrease blood pressure, reduce symptoms of depression and anxiety, and improve physical conditioning by accumulating small bouts of physical activity throughout the day.

Research tells us people are more likely to increase physical activity and continue when exercising ten minutes, three times a day, rather than thirty minutes all at once. The three ten-minute segments produce nearly the same results. Are you feeling excited about the possibilities? Think about chores, activities at work, and your hobbies. Climbing stairs, vacuuming, chasing children or cattle, scrubbing floors, making beds, and shoveling snow are all part of your daily exercise. With this in mind, you might take the stairs instead of riding the elevator, walk to lunch instead of driving, or go outside and play. Every movement counts.

The best way to track all this activity is to get a good pedometer. This is the only piece of exercise equipment I use. Eight thousand steps per day is a good day; ten thousand steps is a great day, and twelve thousand steps is super for weight management. This is the best piece of fitness equipment you can own, so buy a reliable, accurate pedometer.

Move a little bit more, a little more often, is a great place to start your mental shift about physical activity. Overcome the urge to save yourself extra steps; instead, look for opportunities to add a few extra steps. Don't apply any minimum or maximum rules, just move a little more often.

Applying This Principle

- Purchase a pedometer. I recommend Accusplit. This device comes in different models, but the basic step counter is all you need. If you follow the Whole Weigh philosophy, you don't need to track calories burned—just your steps.

- Park your car further from the stores or work and add a block when walking the baby or the dog.
- Gardeners, rejoice! All that weeding counts. Add some walking, and you have a well rounded activity program.
- Add a flight of stairs. Take the stairs at work, at home, while traveling, or anywhere else they're available. Every stair counts, up or down.
- Do a ten-minute, moderately vigorous walk, morning, noon and night. You're more likely to do ten-minute walks rather than a thirty-minute workout, and you'll get nearly the same benefits.
- Lift those babies up and down and give them a squeeze—it's a fun weight-training program.

4. Explore the Outdoors

The best way to exercise is outdoors, enjoying the glory of nature. The rhythm of the ocean as waves kiss a sandy beach, the smell of pine along a forest trail, and the silence of snow falling on a winter's evening are gifts to us from God. Our souls awaken in the presence of beauty, and time spent in God's landscape is a form of prayer. The peace and harmony we find outdoors can't be duplicated on a treadmill.

When I owned The Body Garden, a thirty-minute express workout center, a mother of a fourteen-year-old girl wanted to buy her daughter a membership. "She needs to start exercising," exclaimed the mother. Though a membership was at stake, I couldn't help giving this mother the following advice. "Take your daughter to the Black Hills of South Dakota and walk along the Mickelson Trail. It's far more fun, you'll create great lifetime memories and a close relationship with your daughter. You'll find more joy in the outdoors than you will in a gym." I also suggested they do a ropes course or kayaking together—anything they could learn and do together outdoors. Free yourself from the bonds of exercise equipment and instead jump for joy in nature.

Nature is everywhere—and it's free. Every community is blessed with natural treasures. When I lived in St. Catharines, Ontario, I walked along the Merritt Trail and Burgoyen Woods, hiked the

Bruce Trail, and swam in Lake Ontario. As a child living in New York City, I took the train to Rockaway Beach or Central Park and played. Here in South Dakota, I walk in the country alongside rows of corn and cows, hike the Mickelson Trail in the Black Hills, and explore a nearby cemetery—a great place to walk. Find nature right outside your door, and plan day trips or weekend getaways to Mother Nature's best spots. Fill your soul with joy.

I don't recommend using an iPod or MP3 player outdoors, because it robs you of the spiritual connection to nature. Music is great for the gym, but when outdoors, allow nature to speak to you.

Applying This Principle

- Try something new and don't let fear, or your body, stop you. Rent a kayak, take a ropes course, learn to fish, golf, surf, or scuba dive. Be bold and brave.
- Explore all the places in your community that offer spaces for physical activity. This could include walking trails, Frisbee golf, horseshoes, golf courses, hunting, cross-country ski trails. Choose a new park each week to explore.
- Book an adventure vacation. Try a cattle drive, whitewater rafting, a horse pack trip, or an archaeological tour. The website www.gordonsguide.com offers fabulous tips for outdoor adventure tours.
- Find a spot in your community that connects you to the serenity of nature. Gaze at the stars from a roof, walk in the rain or snow, listen to crickets at dusk, and ponder a beautiful garden. "The best things in life are free," goes the song.

5. Work Out

Surviving a tough workout can make us feel great. The music blares, you gasp for air, your muscles burn, and the taste of salt crosses your lips. You pray it will be over, and when it ends, you're exhausted and exhilarated.

This type of workout most often happens inside a health club, in a spin class, boot camp, toning, circuit training, or a host of other vigorous programs. The energy of music, clanking weights, and encouragement from a trainer or instructor can get you working to the max. Ohhhh—it feels so good to be done.

If you choose this type of physical activity, I offer this advice: Do it because you love the feeling you get when it's over—that satisfying workout high. If you approach a workout with the same old motives; "I've got to lose weight, burn calories and fat, and tone up," then you're focused on extrinsic results and not intrinsic fun. This is temporary motivation, and the results will be temporary. Work out because you love the action, the hard work, and the high you get when you're done. That's why you do it—because it feels good.

When friends recommend a fitness class or program, they share their excitement about a great instructor, the moves, the music, and the dynamics of the class, not how many calories they burned. I attended my first Zumba class with Tammy, my step-daughter-in-law. I love dancing, so Zumba appealed to me. I was delighted I could do all the dance moves and complete the workout. Never once during class did I think of giving up or wonder how many calories I was burning. I concentrated on the moves, felt the energy of the instructors and the music, and was surprised when class was over. Why would I attend another Zumba class? The music, the moves, the dance, the rhythm, the hooting—it pumps me up. I have fun! The more I focus on the intrinsic motivators, the more likely I am to continue. I would do it even if I never lost a pound.

Workouts are everywhere, in different styles. Explore until you find the right facility, class, instructor, or personal trainer. You should feel good when it's over. Commit to the workout, love your body, and go for the burn.

Applying This Principle

- Know yourself and whether a good workout at a gym is the right choice for you. Don't do it because you are trying to lose weight. Do it because you enjoy the workout.
- Visit different facilities and get a free trial, class, or short-term membership before committing to a long-term membership.
- Consider a facility with 24-hour privileges if you need flexibility in your life.
- Hint: Wear compression/spandex clothing under your loose-fitting workout clothes. You'll work harder.

- Experiment with different classes and instructors until you find one that pumps you up.
- If you're doing repetitious cardio machines, get your iPod or MP3 player going. Music helps you work out longer. Watching TV won't do that for you.
- Challenge yourself beyond your perceived limits on the cardio machines. On alternate days double-up your workout. Surprise yourself.

6. Move and Meditate

I watched a lovely film nearly twenty years ago, called *Meditation in Motion.* A woman stood atop a hill doing tai chi, while a gentle breeze rustled through the trees. The film was promoting the practice of tai chi, a contemplative martial art that combines the mind, breath, and movement to create a calm, natural balance of energy. I was mesmerized by the film and struck by the contrast of peaceful tai chi movements, versus a high-energy aerobics class. Since I've always had a strong belief in mind-body integration, I related to the benefits of contemplative movement.

Yoga and tai chi are the most notable mind-body movement techniques. Each offers a variety of styles, and each rooted in ancient cultures. Tai chi comes from China, and yoga from India. These methods reflect centuries of accumulated wisdom before the advent of modern medicine. They work in harmony with the body, the mind, and chi—the body's internal energy—to achieve balance, healing and health. North American exercises focus on using muscle energy for cardiovascular fitness, caloric expenditure, and health. Both styles give us health benefits, achieved in different ways.

I recommend experimenting with meditative exercises to gain the benefits of body-mind-energy integration. As these exercises heighten body awareness and quiet the mind, they also improve muscular balance, strength, and flexibility. Focusing on the breath teaches our wandering minds to experience the moment. Attention to breathing and the sensation of moving into and out of poses heightens the connection to internal energy and promotes a feeling of wholeness.

Other helpful practices that build on mind-body integration include Pilates, Nia Dance, Alexander Technique, and Feldenkrais's Method. Some of these programs are rooted in therapeutic movement that evolved to be suitable for the general population. They all claim to help with increased body awareness, muscle toning, postural benefits, increased flexibility, and mental calmness. Each is different, and all are excellent. They engage the entire being—a delightful way to find balance and grow in good health.

Applying This Principle

- Release the idea that effective exercise must be vigorous and sweaty. A quiet mind may be all you need. Move gently even while walking, and tune in to your breath and movements.
- Walk in a peaceful place (I go to our beautiful cemetery), and walk tall. Feel your spine lengthen and imagine an angel is making your body and steps light. Focus on something in the distance. Be aware of your breath. Meditate.
- Rent a DVD of tai chi or yoga and try a sequence of movements for at least four weeks. You may get hooked.
- When doing any physical activity, including swimming, running, and cycling, focus on body awareness. Sense the energy of the movement as it travels through each muscle and joint.
- As you read this, extend your arm to the side perpendicular to the floor, as a dancer would, one joint at a time, or think of throwing a baseball. Feel the energy travel from your shoulder and through each joint until it reaches your fingertips. That's body awareness. Do the same while walking or performing any form of movement.
- Know yourself. You may respond to vigorous dance programs like Nia, or prefer the more gentle movements of yoga and tai chi.

Chapter 10

Whole Weigh Thinking

"Our life is what our thoughts make it."
— *Marcus Aurelius, Roman Emperor*

In this chapter I offer several guidelines to help you adjust your thinking so you see yourself and your journey in a more positive light. Years of chronic dieting left deep neural pathways in your brain that say you are weak, unworthy, and ugly with fat. But they are not true. That is why you can never diet again. Another diet failure will only strengthen those nasty beliefs. Where do those beliefs get you? It is time to reroute your thoughts down a happier road. Never diet again; think good thoughts, and realize your magnificence.

There is mounting scientific evidence that your thoughts and beliefs have a powerful impact on your physical and mental health. What we believe is what we get. While I am guessing you agree with this statement; the problem is most of us do not intentionally utilize the power of our thoughts to produce positive outcomes. Instead, we allow our emotions to dictate our thoughts, making them situational and not intentional thoughts. This is true for positive or negative thoughts; unfortunately, negative thoughts have dominance, but positive thoughts have more power.

When you get on the scale and discover you have not lost or have gained weight, your negative emotions prosper. This triggers negative thoughts, "I'm miserable and depressed. I hate my body. I hate myself. I have no willpower." With repeated failures, these messages became entrenched, literally. They form deep neural pathways, and they're easier to generate. This belief is transmitted to every cell in your body, and your cells respond. You feel despair, hopelessness, pessimism, so you binge and give up hope.

With deliberate intention, you can change your thoughts and beliefs, and if you're consistent, you can change your biology. You'll form new neural pathways in the brain. Prayer, meditation, and affirmations are the mental conduits to more positive thoughts and beliefs, but so are charitable acts, expressions of gratitude, and love. Fill your brain with goodness and love, and your mind and body will begin to heal.

As a chronic dieter, your positive thoughts and emotions may be stifled and not easy to elicit. So, it does require some effort to overcome the urge to feel sorry for yourself. But you must commit to this effort. Your thoughts have power. We know this from research on the *placebo effect* used in research studies. In drug research trials, some people get the drug treatment and others get a sugar pill, called a placebo. Both groups improve, and in some cases, the people taking the placebo do better. They simply believe they are getting treated and feel better even though they are taking a blank pill. The numerous examples of this type of research is staggering, all pointing to the simple truth that what you believe is what you become. Let me repeat that statement; what you believe is what you become.

Believe the following statement, for it is the truth.

> You are an extraordinary human being. There is only one like you. You are blessed with special gifts, talents, and insights. You have all you need to fulfill your dreams. You are whole, you are full of grace and you are ready to step into your best life.

This is the message you must carry in your heart. Be kind to yourself and recognize your magnificence. See the best of life, the best of love, and the best of everything.

What follows are guidelines reflecting the current research in positive psychology and messages from spiritual and philosophical writers and leaders. These guidelines will help you think good thoughts more often, boost your positive emotions, expand your good energy, and get you feeling good about yourself—a primary ingredient for vibrant health and wholeness. Be intentional and not situational—practice the power of thinking good thoughts each day.

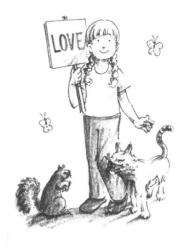

What you <u>believe</u> is what you get.

1. Think Good Thoughts

Your thoughts generate mind maps—pathways of thinking you follow each day. When you feel hopeful, your thoughts select mind maps that lead to high mountains where you see all of life's possibilities. When you're miserable, your thoughts follow mind maps that lead to the basement of life, where you feel trapped and lonely. What you think about comes about. So, I offer this suggestion: think good thoughts, and good things will come about.

Earlier in the book I described my husband's heart attack and bypass surgery. As I wrote this section a year later, he was facing prostate cancer. Naturally, the news of his cancer triggered strong emotions in me: fear, frustration, guilt, sadness, worry, and stress. I thought about the situation in the following ways:

- "It isn't fair having this happen when we live such whole, healthy lives."

- "If I hadn't minimized my husband's symptoms, this wouldn't have gotten so serious. I feel responsible."
- "What if my husband becomes incontinent, the cancer has metastasized, or he needs chemo? Our lives will be complicated, and he might even die."

Negative thoughts like these come unbidden, and they're difficult to overcome. At this juncture I need to make choices. Which mind maps will I choose—hope or fear? Which mind maps will benefit my husband and his care? Which thoughts will encourage the best outcome? The answer is obvious. I need to think good thoughts. I can't fret about the past, because it's over and the future is yet to be told, so why worry about the "what ifs"? I need to focus on the present. What do I know is true at this moment?

- My husband is generally healthy, so he'll do fine.
- We're fortunate to live near the Mayo Clinic in Rochester, an amazing place.
- We have a loving relationship with each other and our family. This crisis will bring us closer.
- I'm nearly finished with the book, so I'll have lots of time to devote to his recovery.
- Most of all I'm grateful for my husband and the way he thinks. He accepts life's hardships as moments in time in the journey of life. He sees no value in worry. "This is life," he says. "Just keep stepping forward."

The change in my thinking about this situation from negative to positive wasn't instantaneous. Once I made a deliberate decision to be more positive and find things that were right, I began making the transition. It took a few hours to shift from fear to hope. In the past I might have needed days or weeks, but my personal commitment to thinking good thoughts more often had built up my positive emotional bank account, so the transition came more quickly.

I'm pleased to report he had an incredibly positive outcome from the surgery, so all is well. I do believe lots of positive affirmations, prayers, energy healing, and meditation contributed to the positive outcome. The healing atmosphere of the Mayo Clinic and of course our brilliant doctor, Dr. Karnes, a model of positive energy, boosted my husbands prognosis and recovery.

Barbara Fredrickson, the author of *Positivity,* emphasizes throughout her book that positive emotions accumulate and multiply. The more you experience positive emotions, the more resilient you become, making it easier to put the brakes on negativity and bounce back from hardships. [29] Your life will flourish if you make a deliberate intention to choose and pursue positive emotions more often.

The phrase, *think good thoughts,* is a gentle reminder to see things with a more positive frame of mind. When negative thoughts begin to invade, reconsider. Like your computer, click on the search icon and scan for good thoughts about any situation. Marci Shimoff , in *Happy for No Reason,* offers a realistic suggestion. Don't force a positive thought that you may not fully believe in that moment, instead "lean into it." "When you lean into a happier thought, you're not trying to convince yourself of anything. You're simply shifting your focus from a part of the situation that makes you feel bad to a truthful part of situation that makes you feel better."[30]

As an example, take the thought: "I hate myself for eating so much food. I feel so stuffed." Lean into the shift with a more truthful thought. "The food I ate was delicious and thank heavens I don't stuff myself all the time." Be deliberate about committing to the shift, but be kind to yourself and lean into it. It takes effort to dial down despair or anger and tune in hope. Do it in small incremental steps until you begin to feel the shift. It does get easier over time, and you do feel your positive emotional bank account growing, making the next time you are searching for positive thoughts a little easier.

29 Fredrickson, Barbara. 2009. Positivity. New York: Crown Publishing.
30 Shimoff, Marci. 2008. Happy For No Reason. New York: Free Press. p. 114.

Applying This Principle

- Be deliberate about thinking good thoughts when you are feeling negative emotions. Allow yourself to experience anger, frustration, and sadness, but sooner than later, transform your thoughts and begin to see benefits, advantages, and opportunities that arise from negative situations. Difficult situations are often the trigger for positive personal growth.
- Banish what you believe others might think about you. It does not matter what others think—it only matters what you think.
- For a few minutes each day, read inspirational words from a book, a calendar, or an inspiring website, listen to a CD, watch a DVD, or go to www.youtube.com and search for inspiration. It's a positive way to start your day.
- Check out your belief system. Do you generally see the world and all people through a negative or positive lens? Do you wallow in the negativity of life, or do you rebound quickly and see possibilities? Do you tend to focus on the issues of life rather than glories of life? A positive lens brings richer rewards and less strife.
- Watch funny videos, anything that makes you laugh, and when you do, negative emotions will fade away.

2. Ask, "What Did I Do Right Today?"

Ask the simple question "What did I do right today?" and you begin to change the way you think. As a chronic dieter, you're adept at recognizing all the mistakes you make on your quest to become thinner. You may even record and analyze those mistakes. Forget that nonsense; it keeps your inner critic alive. Fuel your inner champion by recording and analyzing the things you do right each day.

At the fitness center I once owned, we held team competitions for weight loss, something I now regret. Why? The focus was on pounds, which perpetuates the Chronic Dieters Fatigue Syndrome. I knew this, but did it anyway with the excuse that a weight loss competition would bring people in the door. It brought new members in, but I handed them another weight loss failure—weight off, months later weight back on.

On weigh-in day, team members presented themselves with much anguish. Before I allowed them on the scale, I asked, "What did you do right this past week?" Invariably, they'd say something like this: "Are you kidding? I had a bad week. My sister got married, and I binged all weekend."

I peppered them with questions, trying to get them to describe the things they did right. This wasn't an easy task, because chronic dieters are cynical and negative about themselves. After much persistence, they would reluctantly pause and think. "Well, I did drink water all week."

"How much?" I would ask.

"Oh, probably three bottles each day."

"Wow," I remarked. "That's great. How much pop did you drink?"

"None," was the answer from one woman who used to consume at least three soft drinks a day.

"So, you didn't drink any pop and instead you drank water. Fantastic!"

This would bring a slight smile in recognition of the fact they'd done something right. But the weigh-in usually ended any feeling of satisfaction. They didn't lose weight, didn't lose enough weight, or gained a few pounds. That's why I advise you not to weigh. You rarely step onto a scale and experience positive emotions, regardless of the outcome.

When you keep track of what you do right, you'll make deposits into your positive emotional bank account. You'll feel happy about the things you do right and begin generating a new idea of yourself. This thinking fertilizes positive thoughts, and begins building a new, more beneficial root system that supports the notion, "I'm okay. I'm doing a lot of things right!"

Applying This Principle

- Train yourself to ask this question: What things have I done today that support my good health and well-being? Everyone does something right each day, more than you think, so don't wimp out and settle for only a few things. Aim to make a list of six to ten things you do right each day for your health and well-being.

- Doing something right includes all the domains of wholeness, so when making a list as suggested above, consider acts of kindness, good thoughts, finished tasks, positive conversations, meditating, prayer, and/or a kind act on behalf of Mother Nature.
- Make a list of all the nutritious foods (those close to Mother Nature) you enjoy eating.
- Write in a journal or spend ten minutes contemplating a time in your life when you felt healthy and good about yourself. Use the following questions to help tell your story.
  - When was it?
  - What were the circumstances?
  - What did you do to bring this about?
  - How did others support your efforts?
  - How did you feel?
  - What things did you do right to help you feel this way?
  - What personal strengths contributed to your success?

3. Be a Gratitude Junkie

Gratitude and appreciation will enrich your life beyond measure. Gratitude is a simple expression of thankfulness, while appreciation is a deep feeling for something of value in your life. In his book, *Thanks*, Robert Emmons, Ph.D., a leading scholar in gratitude psychology, explores how living in a state of gratitude increases our potential for happiness. Along with his colleague, Mike McCullough, Dr. Emmons conducted research to determine the value of expressing gratitude through journaling. The study revealed that people who kept journals of gratitude rather than journals about personal challenges were more optimistic, experienced fewer symptoms of illness, slept better, exercised more regularly, and made improved progress towards personal goals.[31] Who knew gratitude could be such a marvelous tool for health and fitness?

Practicing gratitude as a way of life has gained momentum in recent years. As Emmons says, "The evidence that cultivating gratefulness is good for you is overwhelming." But haven't we known this for thousands of years? Ancient philosophers and theologians

---

31 Emmons, Robert, A. 2007. Thanks. Houghton Mifflin: New York.

promoted thankfulness as a great human virtue, and "Thanks be to God" is part of every religious tradition. So let's heed the wisdom of centuries and be grateful for our blessings.

To truly benefit from the gift of gratitude, make it a state of mind, be generous with your expression of thanks, and reduce your complaining. I firmly committed myself to this state of mind when my resolve was tested during a trip to my sister's home in Scotland shortly after she passed away.

The trip was planned with only a day's notice, so I had a heightened sense of urgency. When I arrived at the airline counter, a supervisor informed me I couldn't board the plane because my transition time between flights in Chicago wasn't long enough and the computer wouldn't accept the schedule. She moved me aside and called the next customer. For the next forty-five minutes, I agonized and pleaded with the woman, but she refused to help me. Desperate, I called Orbitz, where I'd booked the flight. They tried to help, but the airline employee refused to give me a boarding pass. She revealed that she hated Orbitz, and then I knew she had no intention of helping me. Her shift ended, she left, and a baggage loader arrived to finish up a few late travelers. I tearfully explained the situation and in a matter of minutes he overrode the computer and handed me a boarding pass. At that moment, I decided to thank everyone who helped me instead of complaining about the one person who stonewalled me.

I encountered many more obstacles during that long day and night, but I made every connection, thanks to assistance from wonderful people. I sincerely thanked each person along the way and followed up with letters for those who went above and beyond. In Chicago, where I had little time to catch my next flight, Antonio of Air Canada parted a sea of people so I could run to make my connection. In addition, he upgraded me to a first-class ticket for my flight to Scotland. What a bonus! I believe my state of gratitude unleashed the genuine power of human kindness.

I felt a shift in my spirit when I consciously made a decision to focus on gratitude. I noticed people's efforts to help instead of focusing on those who stood in the way. I felt less agitated with circumstances beyond my control, like weather and plane delays. This was a powerful lesson in the benefits of gratitude.

Gratitude is now my way of life—a source of joy and happiness. I write many notes of thanks, acknowledge great service, and resist the urge to complain. When I occasionally complain about a service or an error, I do so with a tone of respect.

Dr. Martin Seligman, the father of positive psychology and a professor at University of Pennsylvania, devised a brilliant assignment at the suggestion of one of his students. They held a Gratitude Night. Students brought a guest to class whom they wished to thank for being important in their lives. The students expressed their gratitude through well-planned testimonials. The whole class cried. Gratitude Night is now the highlight of his positive psychology class at the university.

Dr. Seligman states in his book, *Authentic Happiness*, "Insufficient appreciation and savoring of the good events in your past and overemphasis of the bad ones are the two culprits that undermine serenity, contentment, and satisfaction."[32] Be a gratitude junkie; you'll experience more life satisfaction, feel more optimistic, sleep better, and exercise more regularly. This is a simple strategy to implement, so start now.

If you choose gratitude as a way of life, the benefits are enormous. Begin a daily ritual of counting blessings and showing appreciation for others. Good feelings will resonate, and you'll build interest in your positive emotion bank account—your source of resiliency. Remember the old saying, "What goes around comes around."

Applying This Principle

- Keep a gratitude journal or take a moment each day to silently acknowledge things for which you are grateful. You can include simple things, such as a warm home in winter, a walk in the woods, or a treasured gift. Don't overlook things that are troubling you, for within each of those troubles lies insight and a special gift just for you. (See Appendix I)
- Read *Authentic Happiness* by Dr. Martin Seligman, and duplicate his Gratitude Night described above and on page 74 in his book. He encourages you to write and share a testimonial with someone who is important in your life.

---

32 Seligman, Martin, E.P. 2002. Authentic Happiness. New York: Free Press. p. 70.

- Stop and smell the roses, as the saying goes. Consciously acknowledge and offer thanks for moments when nature, art, and music resonate within you.
- Write letters of gratitude for exceptional service, rather than letters of complaints for bad service.
- Right now, sit down and make a list of ten people you need to thank. They may have comforted you in a time of need or been your best cheerleaders. Maybe they shared a meaningful experience with you or complimented you in a way that made you feel good. Whatever the reason, write a simple note of thanks. Make this practice a habit.
- Take every opportunity to genuinely thank people who serve you daily: wait staff, bus drivers, store clerks, receptionists, bank tellers, cashiers, and others.
- List ten things you appreciate about a parent, spouse, child, or sibling. Let it resonate and feel the love and appreciation. Then, try this for someone from whom you are estranged. Feel your love and appreciation grow.
- Say grace before each meal, even if only a small, silent prayer.
- List ten qualities about yourself that you truly appreciate and for which you are grateful. You may struggle, but do not stop until you have ten.
- List ten things you appreciate about the current circumstances in your life.

4. Be Affirming

I was slow to buy into the benefits of self-affirmations. I felt they were fairly silly. "Look into the mirror and tell yourself you are wonderful. Are you kidding?" As my personal journey unfolded I realized how critical affirmations were to transform your negative thoughts to positive ones. I finally made the connection after I read books like Wayne Dyer's *Power of Intention*, Lynne McTaggart's *The Intention Experiment*, and *Ask and It Is Given* by Esther and Jerry Hicks. From these books and others, I learned that my beliefs about myself originate within my own thoughts. What you think about yourself becomes true, even though you may not believe it.

"I'm so uncoordinated."

"I'm directionally challenged."

"I'm an emotional eater."

"I'm too old."

"I can't walk that far; I'm too heavy."

"I'm not very athletic."

You adopt behaviors to confirm your beliefs because your mind won't allow you to lie to yourself. You demonstrate and call attention to your clumsiness, your age, and your disease, so your belief and behavior are consistent.

This is illustrated by the story about cooking I shared earlier in the book. "I hate cooking and I'm not good at it." My actions confirmed these words, because I needed to be consistent with my own belief. I never looked for or followed recipes, avoided cooking whenever I could, rarely invited friends over for dinner, and always joked with my friends that I hated cooking. All these patterns of behavior confirmed my belief, "I hate to cook."

My niece Laura, a gourmet cook, challenged me on my statements about cooking after I lectured her on the power of thought. At that moment I changed my thoughts from "I hate cooking" to "I like cooking and I'm good at it." My actions now reflect those thoughts. I cook often, and I'm more willing to experiment with recipes.

As a chronic dieter, you've created distorted truths about yourself. You've adopted behaviors and actions that confirm these truths. You eat when you're emotionally charged because that's what you believe you do. You only walk a short distance because you believe you're too old to go any further. You binge eat because you're convinced you lack will power.

Many chronic dieters share another, more subtle belief: our weight defines our sense of worth. Deep within your psyche, you say, "I'm too fat to be worthy of unconditional love." Now, you must act in ways that support the belief. Your spouse says, "I love you," but you secretly doubt it because you're fat, so you timidly ask, "Are you sure you love me?" Your spouse, feeling slightly annoyed because you continually ask this question, replies, "Of course I love you, but you don't seem to believe me." You feel sorry for yourself and you're certain he/she can't love you completely, because you're fat.

You tell yourself, "I know my spouse wishes I was thinner, so he/she can't really love me." You then critique every move and word your spouse utters, looking for confirmation that, in fact, he/she does not love you. You challenge your spouse on the notion of love, you minimize a compliment, or you go off somewhere and pout. All your behaviors confirm your belief that you aren't worthy of being loved, while in fact your belief is a lie—your spouse truly loves you. This is a sad outcome of chronic dieting.

Replace negative affirmations with positive thoughts, and then do things to support these new beliefs:

"I enjoy cooking."

"I eat light as a bird."

"I love going for early morning walks."

"I have a fantastic, healthy body."

"I'm full of energy."

"I have a wonderful spouse who loves me unconditionally."

Positive affirmations seed and fertilize your brain with beneficial thoughts that lead to positive behavior. The Law of Attraction is built upon this premise: what you think about comes about.

Experience Your Good Now and *You Can Heal Your Life* by metaphysical teacher Louise Hay is filled with beautiful self-affirmations. Louise tells us, "When we really love ourselves, everything in our life works." She explains that excess weight and other physical ailments stem from the common fundamental belief, "I'm not good enough." Louise states, "Diets do not work. The only diet that does work is a mental diet—dieting from negative thoughts."[33] The affirmations inside her book help readers overcome self-criticism, resentment, and guilt. Please read Louise Hay's books. You'll gain the tools to feel better about yourself.

Applying This Principle

* Buy the book *Experience Your Good Now* and *You Can Heal Your Life* by Louise Hay and use her inspiring affirmations to help

---

33 Hay, Louise L. 2008. You Can Heal Your Life. Carlsbad, CA: Hay House Inc. p. 9.

you banish self-criticism. Every chronic dieter needs to own at least one of these books.

- Sign up for an online daily affirmation service.
- Write a brief self-affirmation designed to combat your personal demons. Have it laminated and placed where you can see it often and recite the phrases.
- Become ritualistic about your self-affirmations. Every morning when you look in the mirror, recite a simple affirmation. This may seem odd at first, but the thought will eventually resonate and help change negative behavior.
- Add short affirmations to the vision statement you created in Chapter 7. Keep them on your computer and cell phone, where you'll read them daily.
- Take up the call of Caitlin Boyle, editor of *Operation Beautiful*, and place post-it notes in public places with the words, "You are Beautiful". This is a wonderful kick-start for self-love and appreciation. www.operationbeautiful.com

5. Be In the Moment

A photograph captures a couple's warm embrace, a soft smile of an aging parent, and the angelic face of a sleeping newborn. These images represent moments in your life that are worth treasuring. As you gaze upon the photographs, your attention is focused; you are in the moment, just as you were when the picture was taken. Being *in the moment*, sometimes referred to as mindfulness, means having an agreement with yourself to give attention to the present moment. The benefits are enormous, but this gentle practice isn't as easy as you might think.

The past and the future are the sources of our worries and can occupy a good part of our daily thoughts, neither of which is based in the present moment. The past, of course, is done; we can't change it, so why fret? The future is unpredictable, so it's pointless to worry about something that may not happen. Then consider all the small things we fret about; I don't like this color; I should have bought the blue one; and I don't know what will happen if he doesn't come. These types of thoughts clutter our minds each moment of every hour of the day. It's a waste of mental energy.

Mindfulness suggests your thoughts and feelings need to stay in the present moment. Using your senses, focus your attention on your movements, sensations, and surroundings without judgment. In practice, you sit down to eat and allow your mind to savor the food with all your senses. Your attention is on the experience of eating and not the project you have to get done before the end of the day. Or, you walk through the park and notice the smells and sounds of nature. You're aware of your body's sensations as you place your feet on the earth beneath you. You feel the air flowing across your face as you look up and see the blue sky. This is how to be "in the moment." Your mind is not fretting about a comment you wish you hadn't made, or the outcome of an upcoming event. If you stay with the present moment you will find peace and tranquility, even on a bad day.

In the past, during a conversation with another person, my mind would flit from one thought to another. I would politely nod, but my brain was in another zone. As I began understanding the concept of being "in the moment," I made it a personal priority to be present in all my conversations. Now, during conversations, I listen intently and gently push aside any thought that competes for my attention. Until I made this conscious effort, I never realized how distracted I could be from the present moment. I also didn't realize how much time I wasted worrying unnecessarily. If I were late for an appointment I would fret: "I should have left earlier." "What will they think?" "It's so impolite." "I'm so bad about time." These thoughts are such a waste of energy. If I am late, so be it; what will be, will be. Worrisome thoughts will not help me.

Once I allowed myself to experience the moment, calmness moved in. I noticed my body wasn't racing in idle, and my mind gently hugged the present. I discovered the pleasure and peace of being in tune with the moment—the now.

This practice has improved my sleep. I used to awaken during the night, at least twice a week, besieged with worry. My husband always asked, "What are you thinking about?" When I told him my tangled thoughts, he followed with, "Think sleep." His advice is always so simple. He's right; it's all a matter of thinking or not thinking. I will fall asleep, if I stay in the present moment and don't fret about the past or future. My strategy is to deliberately concentrate on the rhythm of my breathing, the beating of my heart, and the sensations of my body in communion with my husband's. Mmmmm, that's a moment worth being in. Why would I want to spend time worrying when I can relish my body cradled next to my husband? Thoughts of future events and circumstances can wait until tomorrow as I slip into a blissful state of sleep.

What does all this have to do with weight and health? I used to fret while slicing vegetables for a salad, thinking of other things I could be doing. If I were on a diet that required certain food preparations, I tended to feel self-pity or resentment, so I rarely enjoyed the preparation. Now, being in the moment, I relax, focus and take pleasure in slicing vegetables and preparing food for a healthy meal, without any thoughts of future or past moments.

The same applies to my walks. While walking, I think less about things I need to get done and more about the moment, fresh air, and the stillness of morning. I'm aware of my movements and feel a communion with my surroundings. I don't distract myself with music; I want to be in harmony with nature, my body, and my inner awareness. Walking is no longer a chore; it's more like a quiet meditation.

A quiet mind is one of the greatest benefits of being in the moment. During most of my adult life, I thought a constant stream of thoughts was my greatest asset. My brain was constantly at work analyzing, critiquing, learning, researching, evaluating, and creating. I believed everyone should do more thinking—it's a vital part of living. Now I realize too much thinking is debilitating. I over-analyzed most things, which often led to brain freeze. Then, I would shut down and do nothing. Not much forward progress can happen that way. With so many thoughts filling my brain, I was deaf to my inner wisdom and the voice of God. Now I appreciate a quiet mind that brings peace, creative expression, and a connection to the Divine Source.

I consider myself a novice at being in the moment. I'm still deliberate with my intentions, but I persevere because the benefits are so clear. I urge you to become a student of this practice. Be in this moment. Allow yourself to become intimate with the words on the page of this book. Ponder their meaning. Over time, the benefits will reveal themselves. Your mind will be still and inner peace will enrich your life.

Applying This Principle

- Read Eckert Tolle's book *The Power of Now,* or *Wherever You Go, There You Are* by Jon Kabat-Zinn. These and other books on mindfulness will help you understand the extraordinary power of the present moment.
- Begin the practice of being in the moment by starting with one short activity you perform each day, such as making a bed, cleaning your eyeglasses, or brushing your teeth. Become totally aware of every movement and sensation. Do not think about, just sense it.
- While practicing being in the moment, don't try to force your mind to be without thought—gently guide it back when it wanders.
- Use breath as your beginning point when trying to practice being in the moment. Take in one deep breath and recite as you inhale, "I am in the moment"; do the same when you exhale. This simple ritual will guide your mind to the present moment.
- Focus your attention and use all your senses as you prepare a meal. Feel, smell and see the rich colors and textures of the food and all the utensils you use in preparation. Notice how this relates to "savor the flavor" in Chapter 8.
- While moving, become aware of all the movements and sensations; your muscles, joints, arms swinging, and the flow or air as you breathe. Stay focused on body awareness during your walk, workout, or adventure; I promise it will fire up your motivation.
- Use your senses as a stimulus for being in the moment. Check in with each sense: sight, smell, hearing, touch, and taste.
- Mindfulness takes practice, so be patient with yourself. You will become more aware of the practice and do it more often.

6. Be Inspired

When you're inspired, you're filled with a desire to act, think, and behave in ways that move you closer to your best self. You have clarity, energy, and an urge to do something extraordinary. This is not the infomercial that urges you to call now and purchase the latest exercise craze. That's not inspiration, that's marketing psychology at work. Inspiration is positive energy and moves through the soul. Your spirits are lifted and you feel a shift—a change in the way you see yourself. You want to make a difference in your life and the lives of others.

Your vision statement is a source of inspiration. It brings you clarity and describes you at your best. The more you recite it, the more it fills your soul and body—you feel inspired to be your best. All things with a positive energy will inspire you. It could be a powerful true story of someone who triumphed over adversity, or something simple, like the sight of a rainbow at a moment of despair. These stories and moments fill you with good energy.

All things have energy with a negative or positive vibration. With this in mind consider the simple choices you make each day that positively or negatively affect you. TV shows, news programs, movies, books, magazines, music, art, and even conversations can influence your mood and level of inspiration. Each one of them emits energy—negative or positive. I have significantly reduced the time I spend watching news. I once had a big appetite for journalism programs on politics and crime. I would get agitated and angry, producing lots of negative energy. I had to stop it. I knew negative energy was bad for my body, soul, and mood. Now I watch cooking shows, *Extreme Home Makeover*, *Amazing Race*, and *Sunday Morning*. I limit myself to a half-hour of evening news. My iPod is filled with uplifting music, and my movie choices are based on fun entertainment or an inspirational message.

I also have minimized my participation in negative conversations. Gossip and wallowing in others' misfortunes is bad energy. I excuse myself from gossip or redirect the conversation when I can. This is a practice and sometimes I struggle, but I know I feel better and benefit from conversations of hope and inspiration.

All of my personal daily rituals are meant to increase positive energy and my daily inspiration. I begin my day by contemplating my vision, then I read the daily message from *The Power of Intention* flip calendar by Wayne Dyer. With this simple ritual I know I'm more likely to think and act in ways that move me closer to the best version of myself. Later in the day, I will randomly choose one of my inspirational books, flip through it, and stop to read a page or two. It always seems I land on a page with the best message for me in that moment. My intention is to feed my brain with good thoughts that will lift my spirits.

Life can be hard some days, so you need to feed your soul and body with positive, inspirational energy. Create beautiful spaces in your home or workplace, free of clutter. Listen to music that lifts your spirits and reduce your viewing of negative television programs. Adorn your home with art, plants, and color. Just do all you can to increase positive energy in your world, and you will be inspired each day to be your best.

Applying This Principle

- Get rid of clutter. Nothing will liberate and inspire you more than less clutter. Do it in small bouts: start by organizing a pile, drawer, file, or closet, fifteen minutes per day. As you build momentum, the task will be easier.
- Fill your home and workplace with natural plants and flowers to brighten your day and freshen the air.
- Create change in your life. Try a new haircut, move furniture, shop in a different store, or paint a room. Change is inspiring.
- Watch uplifting TV programs that leave you feeling good; my favorites are ABC's *Extreme Home Makeover* and CBS's *Sunday Morning.*
- Select movies with inspiring messages. My personal favorites are: *The Pursuit of Happyness, Coach, Patch Adams, A Beautiful Mind, The Blind Side, Erin Brockovich, Remember the Titans,* and *Rudy.* Each of these based-on-a-true-story films tell of perseverance, risk, and personal triumph—good messages for chronic dieters.
- Join Spiritual Cinema to receive a steady flow of inspirational movies, documentaries and short films. View and then discuss the message of the film on the website: www.spiritualcinema.com.

- Select music and books that inspire you. They give off good energy, even sitting on a shelf.
- Excuse yourself from toxic conversations about others, quietly and without judgment or comment. Commit yourself to initiate and engage in positive conversations.

7. Be in Tune to Your Spirit

You're in the car, searching the radio for a station that plays your favorite music and gets clear reception. After a few moments of scanning, you zero in on the perfect station. You settle in and continue the drive, feeling content. Can you guess the analogy here? If you find clear reception and tune in to your spirit, you feel good.

So how do we tune in to our spirits? Meditation is one of the oldest and most effective methods. This practice has many forms, so experiment until you find the one that best suits your temperament and lifestyle. I started with Transcendental Meditation (TM). I liked it but only practiced sporadically. As the years passed, I convinced myself I was too busy for meditation; when I did try to meditate, I couldn't sit still long enough. I convinced myself, with my thoughts, that I was not capable of meditating.

It has only been in the past three years that I completely understood the value of meditation and have made a commitment to integrate the practice into my daily life. I know this practice is vital to be in tune with my intuition, my spirit, and Divine Energy. I'm still a novice and not terribly consistent, but getting better all the time.

You may visualize meditation as sitting still for a period of time with eyes closed, reciting a mantra or focusing on your breath as you attempt to banish all thoughts. This is how I meditated at first, and I failed miserably (in my own mind), because I couldn't control the thoughts racing through my head. Then I learned from Eckert Tolle, on Oprah's *New Earth Awakening* Webinar, that when a thought wanders into the mind, we simply acknowledge the thought and let it go. I don't have to resist the thought. I just let it pass through. This simple image changed my meditation practice. I no longer resist thoughts that pop into my head. Instead, I see each thought inside a bubble, acknowledge it, and watch it drift away. This simple adjustment in my thinking made all the difference.

I also gave myself permission to meditate for shorter time periods—five to ten minutes. While writing, I sometimes put my head back and slip into a short meditation as I seek inspiration. I meditate for a few moments in the shower, and five minutes with my face in the morning sun. I also meditate while riding on the back of our Harley Davidson—miles and miles of opportunity for beautiful meditations. Each of these short meditations is a stepping stone toward a more serious meditation practice.

If you find sitting difficult, try meditating with movement, as in yoga, tai chi, walking, biking, or swimming. Focusing on the rhythm of the movements and your breath can be a form of meditation. Another form of meditation in motion is walking a labyrinth—a circular path of several layers leading you to the center of the circle and back to the starting point. Labyrinths have been around for nearly 4,000 years and are associated with most religions of the world, including Aboriginal peoples. They vary in size and structure, but are usually mapped with stones. I recently tried a labyrinth while at the Mayo Clinic and found it to be soothing. Theirs was small, with the design woven into the carpet. Surprisingly, I also enjoyed the finger labyrinth, which you trace with one finger.

Guided meditations create vivid images to aid your focus. For several months I listened to Kathy Freston's CD *The Daily Dose* and found this easier than sitting in total silence. Her voice, the images, and background music really aided my focus, and I became more committed to the practice. I discovered I could sit still and meditate. This experience helped me evolve with my meditation practice.

Prayer is the most common form of meditation. The benefits of prayer are well established in theology, but also validated by research in books like Larry Dossey's *Healing Words* and Lynne McTaggert's *The Intention Experiment*. Prayer usually begins as a conversation with God and often includes a specific focus, such as giving thanks. Prayer seems to be a natural human instinct, so rely on prayer for your meditation if that's what you do best. After you pray, pause to listen, feel, and sense messages from your soul. This is divine communication.

If you still find these practices difficult, first try acknowledging simple forms of meditation you already experience in daily life: quiet reflection in the shower, pausing to enjoy nature's wonders, pondering an inspiring piece of art, or sitting in a quiet room for a moment of peace. Use these moments as portals toward deeper mediation, even if only for a few minutes. Second, be mindful. As I discussed earlier in this chapter, be in the moment. This practice will slow the mind and increase your focus. That's a step forward. Finally, pay attention to your intuition—the internal voice connected to your spirit. Differentiate intuition from ego. Ego will often emit negative energy. Ego will incite you to be angry, jealous, fearful, insecure and defensive. Intuition is positive energy pulling you closer to the wisdom of your soul. Once you connect with intuition, you'll want to listen more often. This will increase your desire to meditate.

Meditation blesses our lives with many benefits, both spiritual and physical. This simple practice can reduce blood pressure and heart rate, relieve stress, and increase energy levels.

The most important benefit is a strong connection to intuition, spirit, and Divine Energy. Such a connection brings calmness and quiet reassurance that we're filled with grace and intimately connected to God. Meditation will quiet the inner critic. Self-criticism comes from the mind-based ego, trying to convince us we'll never be good enough. Drive out those thoughts with meditation and prayer, and allow your spirit to blossom.

Applying This Principle

- Visit the website www.doasone.com to practice conscious breathing. This site is awesome. You can choose the universal breathing, laughter, om, or full spectrum breathing rooms and be with others from all over the world. Each hour they have a special intention such as harmony, oneness, forgiveness or peace.
- If you already practice meditation, then share your stories with others.
- Breathe. If you can't do anything else just breathe for a few moments, paying attention to the rhythm.

- Read Jack Canfield's personal story of meditation in his book, *The Success Principles*. During a seven-day meditation course, Jack had a typical reaction: "The first few days I thought I would go crazy." Then he describes his awakening.[34]
- Introduce yourself to meditation by focusing on being mindful as described earlier. Being in the moment is a gradual step toward adopting meditation as a practice.
- Buy Kathy Freston's meditation CD, *The Daily Dose* at www.kathyfreston.com or www.amazon.com. Her guided imagery is delightful and easy to follow.
- If you're serious about meditation, then go for total immersion by attending a meditation course. This is what Marci Shimoff of *Happy for No Reason*, Jack Canfield, *Chicken Soup for the Soul* and Barbara Fredrickson of *Positivity* all did to advance their meditation. They each tell the story in their books. I plan to attend a meditation retreat before this book is published, and I'll blog about it afterward. Search on the Internet for meditation retreats, or check out the Vipassana Meditation website, where I intend to go.
- Find a labyrinth in your area by going to labyrinthlocator.com. Labyrinth walking is a unique experience and the benefits are many.

---

34 Canfield, Jack. 2005. The Success Principles. New York: HarperCollins. p. 316–317.

Chapter 11

Whole Weigh Living

"You can't cross a sea by merely staring into the water."
— *Rabindranath Tagore, Nobel Laureate for Literature*

Chronic dieters, are you ready? You now have the guidelines for the chronic dieter's recovery program, known as Whole Weigh. Put it all together and you have a way of living. You follow guidelines rather than rules, have healthy relationships with food and with your body, and move in ways that delight your soul.

The primary goal is to feel good about *you*. That's the root of lasting change; no more on again, off again with weight or diets—the symptoms of Chronic Dieters Fatigue Syndrome. You must do something different. Change the way you think about dieting and get on with Whole Weigh Living. With that in mind, I have four more strategies to conclude with: Jump In and Begin, Jump Into Life, Just Breathe and Just Jiggle.

1. Jump in and Begin!

Jump in. Right now do something that moves you forward. Get your vision statement done, use your natural strengths, savor the flavor, go outdoors and play with the kids, write in a gratitude journal. Jump in and do it now—not Monday, not the first of the month, not tomorrow—start right now. You don't even have to get up to do something. Close your eyes, breathe in and out three, times and imagine yourself at your best. Right Now! If you don't do it now, you're thinking too much. Your power is in this moment: Jump in!

Matt Hoover, the winner of the second season on NBC's *The Biggest Loser* lost 154 pounds; some of those pounds have crept back on, but he's maintained a 100-pound weight loss. At a weight he described as chubby, he trained for the 2009 Ironman Triathlon Hawaii. He swam 2½ miles, cycled 112 miles, and ran

26.3 miles. He said two important things in pre- and post-interviews. "I am not thinking like someone who wants to lose weight, I'm thinking like someone who wants to be an Ironman." What is he telling you? It's not about his weight. He's training to connect with his inner power; pushing himself beyond his perceived limits; overcoming doubt and fear. The reward is confidence and self-respect, and if he loses a few pounds along the way, it's a bonus. Following the race, which he finished three minutes shy of an official finish [for an official finish a participant must finish under 17 hours], he said, "It's not about how much you weigh, it's not about what you've done in the past, it's about what you are doing."

What are you doing? Jump in! Do something that makes you feel good. You don't need a program or a plan, and you don't need to journal—you just need to act. Get up and jump ten times, take a hundred steps, eat five grapes, drink a glass of water, breathe in some fresh air. There are no rules. You don't need to do it for thirty minutes or sixty minutes, just move; it all counts.

Eat close to Mother Nature in small portions to nourish your body. You don't have to eat low-fat, sugar-free diet products, just eat foods close to Mother Nature. You could call a friend who inspires you, write a gratitude note, pray, clean a drawer, or listen to music that stirs your soul. Jump in and begin!

2. Jump into Life

The same advice described above is true for other areas of your life: social, emotional, intellectual, vocational, and spiritual. Jump into anything that is in harmony with your true self and leads you to your best life without negatively affecting others.

You've heard the saying "feel the fear and do it anyway"; you've got to take that attitude. Fear is like the *bogeyman* inside your head telling you **not** to jump; it's too scary. These are thoughts generated from your past. Are you going to let a scary thought paralyze your dreams? I understand that fears can be deeply rooted, but remember they are still thoughts that you can banish with new thoughts.

You may not recognize your fears because at times they're disguised. You'll feel cautious and afraid of doing something that would move you toward your dreams, so you stall, ignore, or come up with a silly reason not to advance. I, for instance, have a gregarious personality, so I enjoy meeting new people, networking, and public speaking. But underneath this outgoing personality, I discovered I'm fearful of being detected as incompetent. I don't want anyone to think I don't know what I'm talking about. (Notice, it's related to my natural strengths: my air traits. Competency is a highly valued trait for air people.)

I had a lot of anxiety with essay tests when I was in college and nearly threw up at the thought of people reading my first opinion piece for *Active Living* magazine in Canada. What would readers think about my opinion? Now I know it doesn't matter, but at the time I was a wreck. This hidden fear stalled my dreams. I allowed those fears to rule, and I didn't even know it. The result is I'm sixty-two and completing my first book, when all my life this had been a dream. When I did jump in and started writing, my fears were revealed, and they peeled away layer by layer over the course of four years. The frightening mysteries of writing and publishing are now just steps in a process. Today I feel bold and eager. I expect to write several more books. Please, don't succumb to your fears; jump into life and into your dreams now.

If you need some help understanding your fears, first review your Natural Strengths profile from Chapter 6. Your fears are often related to your personal strengths, core values, and motivations stemming from your personality traits. Secondly, to banish fears, I suggest you read Jack Canfield's book, *The Success Principles.* Over the course of several chapters, he makes fears seem so silly. Jack is also the author of *Chicken Soup for the Soul* series, and he tells the story of how fear tempted him and his co-author, Mark Victor Hansen. The original Chicken Soup for the Soul book was rejected by 144 publishers. That much rejection could have generated intense fear and doubt, but Jack and Mark banished such notions and eventually got published with Health Communications.

Have you ever had fears triggered by just one rejection? I have, but now I recognize how silly it is. Delete the voice of the "bogeyman" in your head.

In *The Success Principle,* Jack poses a simple analogy, a wonderful quality of his writing: he asked if you remember jumping off the diving board for the first time. Anyone who has done it remembers the first time standing at the edge, looking into the water and feeling fearful, but eventually jumping in. That's overcoming fear. We do it all the time: on the first day at work, the first presentation, the first camping trip, the first time skiing—every first was scary, but you did it anyway. You have a track record of overcoming fear. Why be afraid? It's just a thought you created in your head. Delete the thought and jump in.

Our fears engage the emergency brakes while driving in the direction of our dreams. You put your foot on the gas pedal trying to go forward, but there's resistance. Your car trudges forward while it groans from the struggle, but most important you don't advance forward toward your dreams. Release the brakes, jump in, and advance forward. Yes, you may feel foolish, awkward, or unsure. You may even fail a time or two. But you jump in anyway.

Once you commit to jumping in, the emergency brake releases and you'll accelerate toward your dreams. Your courage and confidence grow. Jump in right now: sign up for lessons, enroll in a college course, finish your degree, take a yoga class, join up, become a member, make a call, hire a life coach. Just do something right now, and then tell me what you did and how it feels. Go to www.wholeweigh.com and send me an email describing what you did to jump into life and how it felt.

3. Just Breathe

There is nothing quite as simple and so beneficial as focused breathing. The benefits of taking several minutes, or sometimes just seconds, to focus on your breath are numerous. This simple practice can increase alertness, energize your mind and body, reduce tension and anxiety, calm you down, adjust your mood and help with mental focus. I am suggesting breathing as a coping activity to help you shift your mood, focus, and get you feeling more connected to your internal signals. It's also a great introduction to the more committed practice of meditation.

One of the obvious reasons for all the benefits of deep breathing is the increase of oxygen circulating in the blood. Oxygen feeds every cell, so deep breathing is like a booster breath for the all the body's functions. But it's the rhythmic nature of breathing that makes it so effective and simple—in and out. Right now, focus on the rhythm of your breathing for just three slow cycles while reading the following words: Inhale… exhale… inhale… exhale… inhale… exhale. Do you notice how quickly you are "in the moment" and how easily tension floats away? That's the beauty of focused breathing, in an instant you're induced into a calm place in your mind with less tension in your body. Rhythm, which is a natural sensation in our bodies, makes it easy to transition into a relaxed state.

Take advantage of breathing in all the situations where you may be struggling to make decisions, to get focused or when you're feeling tense, nervous or fatigued. Just breathe! If you're trying to overcome the urge to indulge when you feel full—just breathe! If you're trying to decide whether or not to go for a walk—just breathe! If you can't fall asleep—just breathe! If you're afraid to jump-in—just breathe! Make it a habit. Do it now. Just breathe!

BREATHING TECHNIQUES

1. Technique One: Kinesthetic Breathing 4x4x8

This technique is great for relaxation and mental focus, and can be done anywhere at anytime.

Sit tall and place your right hand near your heart and your left hand on your abdomen. Breathe in through your nose for 4 counts feeling your chest and abdomen expand. Hold your breath for a count of 4. Exhale through your mouth for 8 counts feeling your chest and abdomen deflate. Repeat 3 times.

2. Technique Two: Bellows Breathing 3x15

This technique is stimulating and great for increasing energy and mental alertness.

With your mouth relaxed, breathe in and out through your nose using short rapid shallow breaths. Imagine the rhythm of a bellows used to stoke a fire or a bicycle pump to blow up a tire. Use 2 to 3 cycles of in and out breathing in just one second, and do this for no more than 15 seconds. When you start using this technique you may get lightheaded and hyperventilate, so you may want to start by doing it for 5 to 10 seconds at a time until you get used to it.

3. Technique Three: Relaxing Breaths 4-7-8

This is a great technique to use in a time of frustration and anger or anxiety.

Sit and close your eyes. Place the tip of your tongue on the roof of your mouth. Breathe in through your nose to the count of 4, feeling the abdomen expanding. Hold your breath for 7 counts and then exhale through your mouth with a count of 8, making a sound as the air passes over your lips.

Do As One

There is a marvelous website called Do As One at www.doasone. com which I referred to in the previous chapter. The goal of this organization is to "connect humanity by establishing a legacy of healthy conscious breathing." The website guides you through many different styles and rhythms of breathing.

The visitor to this website can choose from twelve different types of breathing rooms, including the calm breathing room, the activation breathing room, the full spectrum breathing room, and the laughter room. The universal breathing room encourages collective breathing throughout the world at the same time each day. I have a daily alarm on my mobile phone to remind me to participate. There is a world map in each room that identifies the location of the people currently visiting that room. The site is beautiful, simple and very easy to negotiate. One visit and you'll be hooked and sharing this site with all your friends. It is awesome!

4. Just Jiggle

Now it's time to tell you about Just Jiggle, something you do when you're feeling low and your inner critic gets the best of you. This little strategy will shake off the fears, doubts, and negative thoughts that creep up. Your inner critic, which is the voice of your ego, will always be trying to take over, so you must have a strategy to combat it. You can follow many of the suggestions in Whole Weigh Thinking, but there will be times when you falter, start doubting yourself, and convince yourself it's not working; you're destined to be fat. That's all the garbage leftover from traditional diets. When that happens, you must jiggle. I expect you to laugh and think this might be a bit crazy—it is.

I devised this strategy when I was wrestling with my own doubts; my inner critic was trying to score some points and make me feel lousy about myself and my body. I would often say to my husband, "I'm a fraud. I'm writing this book and I'm still fat." "You're not a fraud," he would say. "You're writing this book for people just like you. They need to read about your story and struggles." In my mind, I had to be perfect or I was a fraud. How silly? No one is perfect, so I am in good company.

On one occasion of self-doubt, I had just finished showering and my husband was close by. I stepped in front of him naked and said with anguish, "I have to learn to love this body, just the way it is," and intuitively I started to move in a way that jiggled my fat shouting out, "I love it, I love it. Feel it jiggle, I love it!" I circled around so my husband could see my whole body jiggle. I never let him see my naked bum so this was a moment of real courage. But in that moment, I embraced the idea that my body was worth loving whatever its size. My husband was amused, of course, and giggled gently. Being a bit of an introvert, he just grinned and said, "Shake it, but don't break it, 'cause I love it, just the way it is."

So now Just Jiggle has become a strategy I use to shake off those moments when I feel bad about my body and feel sorry for myself. I jiggle and remind myself my body is awesome and I love it. Sometimes it's just a little jiggle. I jiggle whenever I need to shake off my doubts, love my body, or amuse my husband.

I shared this story with my close friends, and some thought I was nuts. But my dear friend Jeannie got it and helped me during a moment of despair. While my husband was in the hospital for heart surgery, I had a moment when I felt quite low. I called Jeannie with the news, and she sensed my mood. She instructed me to jiggle. I said I would, but she detected my white lie. So she said again, "Jiggle." Jeannie is a wise woman, so I complied. I jiggled, and it worked. I felt a shift in my mood; I smiled and thanked my friend. So now Just Jiggle has a wider application than a method to shake off bad feelings about my body. It helps me shake off many of my negative emotions. It's silly, but sometimes emotional responses to circumstances in life are silly. So, I suggest you shake them off with a jiggle. You can jiggle just one body part, it doesn't matter, the important thing is, just jiggle.

With these four strategies, Jump in and Begin, Jump into Life, Just Breathe and Just Jiggle, you have easy ways for managing life that move you closer toward your dreams. You must be enthused about living the life of your dreams and have ways to shake any doubts. This, after all, is your one and only life. Jump in, breathe, jiggle, and feel good about being *you.*

PART IV

Whole Weigh in Practice

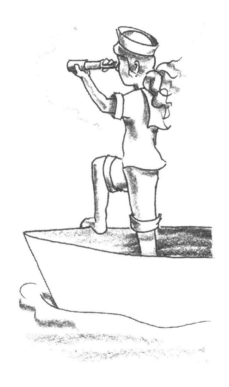

Where you put your
attention
is where you will go.

Chapter 12

The Whole Weigh Checklist

"If you focus on results you will never change. If you focus on change you will get results"

– Jack Dixon, Author

You've finished reading the book or you're taking a peek at the final pages because you're eager to get started, so let's do it. This chapter presents a checklist of all the principles and strategies for Whole Weigh living. Right now, consciously decide to do things in ways you've never done before. You are on a new journey. Rejoice and begin.

There is no perfect way to approach this way of being. Do whatever makes sense to you. But I have made some suggestions to give you focus. Choose a few simple things to practice that resonate with you and begin.

The most important task is to complete your vision statement and/or vision board.

1. Two Things You Need to Buy

1. A journal
2. A good pedometer. I recommend Accusplit.

2. Three Essential Strategies to Adopt

1. Stop diet chatter
2. Wean from weighing
3. Love your body

3. Three Tools You Must Complete

1. **Circle of Whole Being**: Honor yourself as a whole being socially, emotionally, physically, intellectually, spiritually, vocationally, and environmentally. Value and expand yourself

in each dimension, and your wholeness and wellness will grow. Answer the questions at the end of Chapter 5.

2. **My Natural Strengths**: Get to know yourself, your values, your strengths, and your motivations by reading the descriptions in Chapter 6.

3. **Vision:** Create your vision statement and/or vision board as instructed in Chapter 7. You must imagine and feel yourself at your very best. These images are your sources of inspiration that advance you forward. Doing your vision statement and/or vision board is vital for your success.

4. Whole Weigh Principles to Live By

Below are the three primary categories for Whole Weigh Living. You want to begin to integrate these principles into your daily life. This requires focus. Choose three principles to concentrate on for a month. Whole Weigh Thinking is most important, so choose one from Whole Weigh Thinking and two more from any category; thinking, eating, or moving. Choose the strategies that really speak to you and reflect your vision. Don't over think, just feel it and then commit without rethinking your choices. *Jump in, do it, and stay with it!* You can do it. I hope you will keep the other principles in play, but you need a focus to start.

Notice I have not suggested goals, but instead a focus. That is all you need. In the past, you most often have been instructed to select a specific, measurable goal, such as write in your journal five times each week. You will try but often fail, and then you fuel the inner critic. It is best to focus on change using your vision, rather than results. Your vision comes from within and you will grow into it. Remember, you can never fail your vision. So with your vision in mind choose a focus from the three main principles:

1. Eat Close to Mother Nature
2. Go Outside and Play
3. Think Good Thoughts

Whole Weigh Eating

- Eat Close to Mother Nature
  - o Choose foods more often that are close to their natural origin. Reduce the use of packaged, instant, and canned foods. Eat more fresh and organic foods.
- Eat to Nourish Your Body
  - o This is an attitude. The only reason you eat is to nourish your body, so eat only foods that have a nutritional value. Banish the notion that you are an emotional eater.
- Savor the Flavor
  - o Slow down. Use the five "S"s of eating: see, smell, swish, savor and swallow, and avoid drinking while eating. This could be the single most important strategy to implement. It rekindles all your senses while eating.
- Make Water Your Preferred Drink
  - o Choose water more often than any other beverage. Be proud that water is your preferred drink.
- Add a Touch of Color
  - o Add nutrients to every meal with a splash of color. Before you serve or eat your meal, add color with a carrot, radish, pepper, mango, etc.
- Eat a Little Bit Less, a Little Less Often
  - o Reduce all portions by several bites and get used to leaving food on your plate, even if it's only a bite. Eat a little less often.

Whole Weigh Moving

- Go Outside and Play
  - o Play is a great way to get moving: backyard games, tickling, chasing, snowman making, skipping, hide and seek, march in a parade. Every movement counts.
- Do Something Extraordinary
  - o Do something you've imagined but never believed you could do. Run/walk a marathon, take a cycling vacation, swim across a lake or hike a mountain.

- Move a Little Bit More, a Little More Often
  - o Every movement counts, so you can do small bits frequently and still benefit. Do ten-minute walks, ten jumping jacks, run down the block, dance at the wedding, practice yoga for ten minutes, do cannon balls off the diving board, walk the dog, etc.
- Explore the Outdoors
  - o Make a commitment to explore the outdoors. It's brimming with challenges and nature. Hike, explore, treasure hunt, swim, or take an adventure vacation.
- Work Out
  - o Enjoy the routine of a regularly scheduled workout, taking full advantage of classes, trainers, and equipment.
- Move and Meditate
  - o Do quiet, more meditative forms of movement that concentrate on breathing, alignment, and the core muscles of the torso.

Whole Weigh Thinking

- Think Good Thoughts
  - o Gently lean into more positive thoughts and emotions when you're feeling despair and frustration. This will build your positive emotional bank account and you will become more resilient.
- Ask "What Did I Do Right Today?"
  - o Track the things you do right each day for your wholeness, wellness, and health. This switches your focus from negative to positive. This expands your positive energy.
- Be a Gratitude Junkie
  - o Journal or meditate on the things you are grateful for, including people, circumstances, and simple pleasures in your life. This may help with impulse control and increase physical activity. Being grateful generates good vibrations and makes you feel good.
- Be Affirming
  - o Recite positive affirmations so your brain will be rewired to recognize your magnificence. This builds self-acceptance and self-worth and gets you feeling good about yourself.

- Be in the Moment
  - o Be calm and experience the present moment. Right now, as you focus on these words, feel the meaning and don't let your mind stray to things of the past or future. That is worry.
- Be Inspired
  - o Surround yourself with things that lift your soul to a high vibration. Eliminate or at least reduce negative TV, music, or speech. Reduce clutter and add beauty to your surroundings.
- Be in Tune to Spirit
  - o Meditate in any way that brings silence to your mind and soul—guided meditation, moving meditation, silent meditation, and prayer.

Write It Down

From the list above, choose three strategies to focus on for the next thirty days. Choose at least one from Whole Weigh Thinking.

1. _____

2. _____

3. _____

---

5. Journal to Accelerate Progress

Journaling, for some, is a real source of pleasure and, for others, a burden. If you have the urge to journal, then record the things you do right each day. If you're less likely to journal, you can meditate on this for five minutes toward the end of your day. However, for the first couple of weeks, I do recommend you journal as often as you can, to develop the mental practice of recording at least eight to ten things you did right and eight to ten things for which you are grateful. When you just use mental recall, you are more likely to keep your list short. You need to push yourself to come up with a long list so you move beyond the most obvious of behaviors, things, and circumstances.

The two things worth journaling about are:
1. The Things I Did Right Today (See Appendix I)
2. The Things I'm Grateful for Each Day (See Appendix II)

6. Things To Do Daily, Or At Least Often

- Read your Vision Statement or contemplate your vision board often. Let the images resonate within each cell. Feel it, believe it, and be it.
- Journal or mediate on the things you are grateful for in your life.
- Track the things you do right each day to reduce the voice of the inner critic.
- Do simple affirmations to generate more positive vibrations.
- Practice simple breathing techniques described in Chapter 11.

This is the summary of Whole Weigh and you can see it is not difficult, if you are willing to respect your body and nature, God's works of art.

It bears repeating, to be successful you need a focus. I want to repeat one more time, complete your vision. It really is the seed to change your ways of thinking. It will call you forward.

Chapter 13

Whole Weigh Ceremony

"Ceremony marks the time to cast off aspects of yourself and your past that no longer deliver positive results."
– *Lendrick Lodge, Scotland*

Ceremonies mark important moments in our lives: christenings, birthdays, communion, graduations, inductions, marriage, and death. Many of our ceremonies are rooted in religious rites, some for achievement and others marking a passage of time. Ceremonies are very symbolic and seem to be a natural part of the human experience. Something happens to us when we participate or witness a ceremony. Space is opened up within our souls, and a new powerful energy of hope and promise moves in. It marks an ending of one point in life and celebrates the beginning of something new.

If you intend to stop dieting and commit to the principles in Whole Weigh, I recommend participating in or devising your own ceremony. Whole Weigh is a significant shift in your relationship with yourself, your body, and food. You're discarding the old ways of dieting, and instead harmonizing with your body, mind, and soul. Ceremony is the perfect way to symbolize your release from the old ways and the beginning of something new.

Any ceremony you devise needs to symbolically cleanse yourself of negative thoughts and negative energy that years of dieting have inflicted upon you. You could burn or bury symbols of dieting, which could include diet books, diet journals, or calorie counters, or simply put words on a piece of paper indicative of dieting, such as denial, restrictions, fat, or emotional eater. You could also write down those nasty inner critic messages: "I'm not good enough," "I have no will power," or "I hate my body."

The second part of the ceremony needs to symbolize a new beginning and acceptance of the new way of being. You cleanse yourself of the old way and open your body, mind, and soul to a new way. Harmony and wholeness will reign in your heart and soul, and you'll be at peace with your body.

One New Year's Eve, I wrote on several pieces of paper my self-doubts and limiting beliefs—phrases that rattled in my head convincing me, I wasn't "good enough." Then I wrote affirmations to counteract those statements. I placed my self-doubts in a stainless steel bowl, and just before midnight, I went outside in the cold South Dakota night and lit them on fire, declaring myself free of my limiting beliefs. At the stroke of midnight, I took several deep breaths to open up new space for promising beliefs. I waved a smoldering sage and sweetgrass bundle over my entire body beginning with my feet. This was done to cleanse myself of negative thoughts. Then after a few moments of prayer, I recited each affirmation with a deep conviction. After a few more deep breaths, I completed my personal ceremony to free myself of limiting beliefs and replace them with promising beliefs.

I grew to cherish ceremonies during the five years I taught at a Native American University. Smudging ceremonies, like the one I described above, were used often for celebration and during a crisis. Everyone stood in a circle, while an elder went from person to person with the smoldering sage. There was always a deep sense of renewal and a strong connection between my spirit and the Creator.

Ceremonies and rituals symbolize new beginnings and build internal strength. Devise your own ceremony, remembering to cleanse yourself of the past and of your limiting beliefs. Then pray, breathe, and affirm your promising beliefs. Amen.

***

IN CONCLUSION

The purpose of this book was to convince you to stop dieting and love yourself. It is based on the simple premise that you have to change the way you see yourself, before you can change your behaviors. Self-love and acceptance is the source of positive behavior change. The better you feel about yourself the more courage you have to forge ahead and be your best.

Live a healthy and whole life starting today. Fill your heart with love and gratitude, cultivate healthy relationships with others, love and appreciate yourself and your body, eat close to Mother Nature, go outside and play, think good thoughts, jump into life, and when a negative thought invades your brain, breathe in and jiggle.

Appendix I. Samples

The Things I Do Right Each Day

Each day, we all do something right for our health, wellness, and wholeness. Here are some examples of things you may record.

- I engaged in a fun conversation with my children.
- I drank a glass of water instead of pop.
- I overcame the urge to eat a donut.
- I made/ate a great salad with lots of fresh vegetables for dinner.
- I slowed down and savored the flavor.
- I checked in with my body twice today. "Do you want this food?" "Do you want to sit or move?"
- I played with the kids outdoors for twenty minutes.
- I gave a friend a heartfelt compliment.
- I got up ten minutes early and did some Pilates before work.
- I parked the car far away from the store so I could get an extra 200 steps.
- I meditated for five minutes.
- I wrote a note of gratitude for exceptional service.
- I threw out two boxes of stuff.
- I bought some fresh flowers for my home.
- I got a good night's rest.
- I started to read a great inspirational book.
- I got a massage.
- I visited a friend in the hospital.
- I tried a new nutrition-rich recipe today.
- I said a prayer.
- I called an old friend.
- I finished a project.

Appendix II. Samples

The Things I'm Grateful for Each Day

Contemplate the things you are grateful for at least three times each week. Here are some examples you may consider:

- Clean sheets
- The smell of a lilac bush
- A blue sky
- The ability to love and accept all people as they are
- My feet and nose
- The taste of a sweet juicy orange
- A nice compliment from a colleague
- The giggle of a baby
- My new dishwasher
- My sense of humor
- Facebook
- Living in a small town
- My spouse/children/family
- My body and its ability to walk briskly with ease
- My church/social group
- Friendly service where I shop
- The beautiful walking trail
- The color yellow
- The sun on a winter's day
- The sound of the ocean
- Writing skills
- My Smartphone
- My best friend
- My indoor sauna
- My sense of smell
- A swim in a lake/ocean
- The taste of a red pepper

- My heart
- My body
- My morning tea or coffee
- My intellect
- The evening sky
- A shooting star
- The smell of fall
- Children laughing

Appendix III. Samples

Self-Affirmations

I love and accept myself exactly as I am. My body is beautiful and handsome. I am grateful for all my body does to keep me well. I love this body and can feel good health moving through it. Each cell is in sync with my vision to be healthy and fit.

My body relishes movement and moves with ease. It feels alive. I dress my body to express my joy in being who I am. I have nothing to hide. With each passing day I feel stronger and more vibrant. I am in awe of my body's amazing abilities to adapt, heal, and respond to my intentions.

I love my body, I love myself, and I feel good.

~~~~~~

I enjoy cooking wonderful nutritious meals. I can easily follow a recipe and truly enjoy the results of my efforts. It is worth the energy when my family and friends tell me how wonderful the meal was. I feel good about cooking and preparing nutritious meals for my family.

~~~~~~

I appreciate all the gifts God has blessed me with and because of this I love and accept myself.

~~~~~~

I am confident and ready to step boldly into my dreams. It is a wonderful strong feeling with wonderful positive energy guiding me. I love meself and I love my life. From this place I can make a difference in the world.

~~~~~~

I am happy with my life, family and job. I have abundant energy, and a healthy body that moves with ease and thrives on nutrient-rich foods that I savor each day.

~~~~~~

I am an extraordinary human being. There is only one like me. I am blessed with special gifts, talents, and insights. I use those talents to make a difference in the world. I am blessed.

References and Recommend Resources

All of the books and DVDs listed below are ones that I read along my personal journey and in preparation for writing this book. Each one had a lasting effect on me. I want to acknowledge the wisdom and value each of these authors, who fortified my own beliefs with invaluable insights and information. I recommend them to you.

Positive Thoughts and Emotions

Happy for No Reason: 7 Steps to Being Happy from the Inside Out, by Marci Shimoff, Free Press, 2008.
This book is a wonderful source of stories, information and exercises that will help you shift your way of thinking so that "you live from happiness rather than for happiness".

How Full Is Your Bucket: Positive Strategies for Work and Life, by Tom Rath and Donald O. Clifton, Gallup Press, 2004.
This book uses a simple metaphor to highlight the value of positive thoughts and words. It is easy to understand and can be read in one sitting.

Thoughts on Purpose, Thoughts on the Self, Thoughts on Living, and *Thoughts on Relationships*, by Paul Liebau and illustrated by Barry Trower.
These small books of inspiration are absolute gems that capture the theme of healthy thinking and living. They have been part of my life for years, and now part of this book. Order these books at www.liebau.com

The Science and Psychology of Positive Emotions

Thanks: How the Science of Gratitude Can Make You Happy, by Robert A. Emmons, Houghton Mifflin, 2007.
This is an easy to read book on the science and benefits of gratitude.

Positivity: How to Embrace the Hidden Strength of Positive Emotions, Overcome Negativity, and Thrive, by Barbara Fredrickson, Crown Publishers, 2009.
This is the most readable book on the science and practice of positive emotions.

Authentic Happiness: Using the New Positive Psychology to Realize Your Potential for Lasting Fulfillment by Martin Seligman, Ph.D.
An absolute *must read* if you want to understand the true source of happiness and the benefits of positive thoughts.

What the Bleep Do You Know, DVD, Twentieth Century, 2004.
This DVD tells a story while taking you on a scientific and spiritual journey.

Mindfulness

The Power of Now: A Guide to Spiritual Enlightenment, by Eckhart Tolle. New World Library, 1999.
The Power of Now is the book that taught me the relevance and practice of mindfulness in a simple question and answer format.

Affirmations

You Can Heal Your Life, by Louise L. Hay, Hay House, 1999.
A very sensitive and beautiful book, it will help anyone wanting to live their best life.

Experience Your Good Now: Learning to Use Affirmations, by Louise L. Hay, Hay House, 2010.
Affirmations are powerful, and this book is a simple guidebook complete with inspiring illustrations.

Intention and the Law of Attraction

The Power of Intention, Learning to Co-Create Your World Your Way, by Wayne Dyer, Hay House, 2004.
This book launched my journey into understanding the power of thoughts.

The Secret, DVD and book by Rhonda Byrne, Beyond Words, 2006.
This DVD and book is a great introduction into the Law of Attraction and the power of thoughts.

The Astonishing Power of Emotions: Let Your Feeling Be Your Guide, by Esther and Jerry Hicks, Hay House, 2007.
This book helps you to understand the power of your thoughts and emotions with specific references to weight.

The Shift, DVD with Wayne Dyer, Hay House, 2009.
This DVD masterfully weaves three stories of individuals looking for meaning in their lives. Wayne Dyer is the guide that helps them move from ambition to meaning.

The Inner Weigh™, produced and written by Dr. Dave Smiley, 2010.
This DVD speaks directly to the application of the Law of Attraction to weight. It's based on Dr. Smiley's own experience with weight loss.

Spirituality

Anam Ċara: A Book of Celtic Wisdom, by John O'Donohue, Harper, 2004.
The author, John O'Donohue, eloquently teaches the reader to honor the wisdom of the body and soul.

A New Earth: Awakening to Your Life's Purpose, by Eckhart Tolle, Plume, 2005.
This is masterful book, which brings our ego into view and then gently opens space for self and spirit to flourish.

Motivational

Making the Impossible Possible, by Bill Strickland.
If you struggle to fulfill your dreams, you must read this book. It is a gem. You will feel the urge to do something extraordinary when you finish the book.

The Success Principles: How to Get from Where You Are to Where You Want to Be, by Jack Canfield, First Collins, 2005.
Jack Canfield, using concise and common sense language, outlines practical principles for success in any endeavor in life. This book will jump-start any dream.

Food and Physical Activity

Food Matters: A Guide to Conscious Eating, by Mark Bittman, Simon and Schuster, 2009.
Bittman provides a simple explanation about benefits of nutritious wholesome foods and then provides a food plan and recipes to implement a simple way of eating.

Food Rules: An Eater's Manual, by Michael Pollan, Penguin Books, 2009.
This is required reading for Whole Weigh Eating; a super simple set of rules to eat a wholesome diet.

In Defense of Food: An Eater's Manifesto, by Michael Pollan, Penguin, 2008.
"Eat Food, Not Too Much, Mostly Plants." This author points out the dangers of consuming "edible food substances" and the benefits of eating real food.

What to Eat, by Marion Nestle, North Point Press, 2006.
The bible of food, this book answers all the questions related to food including organic foods, bottled water, farm-raised fish, and artificial sweeteners.

The 8 Colors of Fitness: Discover Your Color-Coded Fitness Personality and Create an Exercise Program You'll Never Quit, by Suzanne Brue, Oakledge Press, 2008.
Understand your personal style of fitness based Meyers-Briggs Type® Easy to read and understand.

Self-Awareness

Operation Beautiful: Transforming the Way You See Yourself One Post-it Note at a Time, by Caitlin Boyle, Gotham Press: 2010.
This is a collection of stories of women who left or found post-it notes in public places reminding them that they are beautiful.

Dancing With Your Dragon: The Art of Loving Your Unlovable Self, by Shaeri Richards. Heartfull Productions: 2010.
This book is a beautiful guide to self-love. It's filled with practical examples and simple practices to help the reader expand their awareness.

Me First: If I Should Wake Before I Die, by Betty Healey, Conrad-Jacques Consultants, Inc.: 2009.
This book is the perfect companion to Whole Weigh. The message is, attract the life you desire and step into unlimited personal power.

Fit from Within: 101 Simple Strategies to Change Your Body and Your Life, by Victoria Moran, McGraw Hill, 2002.
The 101 strategies to change your body and your life is a true gem. This is required reading for Whole Weigh fans.

Showing Your True Colors: A Fun, Easy Guide for Understanding and Appreciating Yourself and Others by Mary Miscisin, True Colors, 2005.
Expand your knowledge of your true personality traits using True Colors®.

The Truth about Weight and Obesity

The Spirit and Science of Holistic Health by Jon Robison and Karen Carrier, Author House, 2004.
This powerful book, packed with research, challenges traditional health and weight loss approaches and instead promotes a holistic approach to health. The target audience is Health Promotion Specialists, but anyone can benefit from the information.

Health at Every Size: The Surprising Truth about Your Weight, by Linda Bacon, BenBella, 2008.
If you want to understand the truth about weight and health, you must read this book. It dispels many myths and firmly held beliefs. When you finish reading this book you will have a new relationship with your body, weight, and food.

The Obesity Myth: Why America's Obession with Weight Is Hazardous to Your Health, by Paul Campos.
Campos, with research and great writing, dispels the myths of the traditional fat and diet paradigm, particularly the notion of an ideal body weight as determined by BMIs.

Discover Your Healthy Weight DVD from www.TheBodyPositive.org
Medical professionals explain how dieting ultimately leads to weight gain and health problems. Instead of dieting connect to your inner wisdom and live healthy.

Websites

www.operationbeautiful.com
This site supports the book by the same name. I highly recommend that Whole Weigh readers place "you are beautiful" post it notes in public places. It's great body image therapy.

www.happyfornoreason.com
This is the website for the book of the same name, by Marci Shimoff. There are lots of great resources to help you shift from a negative to more positive state of mind.

www.spiritualcinema.com
Become a member and receive inspirational documentaries and a feature film each month. This is great for shifting your mood and lifting your soul.

www.kathyfreston.com
Order Kathy Freston's meditation tape on this site. I recommend the Daily Dose. It's a great way to learn the discipline of meditation.

www.authentichappiness.com
This site has numerous questionnaires and information on strengths, happiness, gratitude, optimism, work/life balance, and relationships.

www.agapelive.com
This is the site for The Agape International Spiritual Center with the Reverend Michael Beckwith from the film *The Secret*. You can access services through live streaming. It's an awesome experience.

www.doasone.com
This website is a beautiful place to go for moments when you need deep breathing to calm or energize yourself. Their goal is to have one billion people breathe together synchronously by November 11, 2012.

Permission

Paul Liebau and Barry Tower for the quotes and illustrations from the books, Thoughts on Living, Thoughts on Relationships, Thoughts on the Self, and Thoughts on Purpose published by P.S.A. Ventures, London, Ontario, Canada

Acknowledgments

Dear Readers, I am so grateful to you for reading this book; I hope it lightens your journey and you find peace within your soul. We are all worthy. To all the patrons of my services throughout the years in Canada and South Dakota: I want to thank you all for everything you taught me. I often heard, "You should write a book"; it was so validating. Each compliment chipped away at my limiting beliefs until I had the courage to sit with my computer and write.

To my colleagues in Canada, especially FOLP Trainers and those at ParticipACTION: you are the best. I so enjoyed being challenged to learn and grow professionally and personally, with special thanks to Christa Costas-Bradstreet, Dot Bonnefaunt, Pat McKay, Patricia Jackson, Karen King, Connie Jasinskas, Nancy DuBois, Margaret Good, and John Henderson. To the Canadian Active Living Community: you are amazing. I am so grateful I could be a part of such a progressive movement. This includes Joe Taylor, the publisher of *Active Living*, who gave me the opportunity to explore my writing.

The process of writing a book, as I discovered, is a journey of self-discovery. Many times, I would have abandoned this project, but my dear husband Garney Henley wouldn't let me. "Finish the book," he would gently say many of hundreds of times. He believed in me long before I did. He is my life coach and truly my best friend. To each of our children: Dave and Rob, thanks for loving me just the way I am, and Pam, Lori, Jody and Kyle, thanks for your open arms. It takes love and acceptance to feel strong from within.

Angie Nelson, my personal trainer and trusted employee, you were the one who got me started on this book by assigning me the task of writing two pages of my book as a fitness challenge. Brilliant! I need to thank Rita Cook for offering suggestions that shaped this book in the early stages, but more than that, getting me to write with conviction and simplicity. You have some wonderful insights, my friend, and you know me well. Nicole Woolridge, Mickey Scheibe, and Lisa Goglin: each in your own way gave me support to fulfill my dream. Believe in yourself the same way you believed in me. Then there are all the Body Garden members to thank. I am grateful so many of you were open to my ideas and encouraged me to write this book. You taught me my beliefs had merit. I must also thank all my students at Huron University/Si Tanka University. I had so much fun with you all. You opened your minds and allowed my beliefs and points of view to creep in. Physical education is about skill acquisition—and remember no running around in circles to warm-up. Boring!

Marci Schimoff, the author of *Happy for No Reason* and *Chicken Soup for the Woman's Soul*, you gave me a compliment and some encouragement on two occasions: once at the South Dakota Women's Conference and again at the Twenty-First Century Book Marketing Seminar. You need to know your compliment was a booster and your offer of support sent me into overdrive. A sincere compliment can make such a difference. I promise to "pay it forward" in your honor. The same goes for you, Jack Canfield, co-author of *Chicken Soup for the Soul* and *Success Principles*. Our encounter was brief, but you made me believe, with the simplest of words, "Charlotte, you *will* be a best-selling author." Jack's book *Success Principles* had a significant impact on the way I work. I am eternally grateful. Your book is always near. Caitlin Boyle, author of *Operation Beautiful*, what a trip. You are beautiful and so is your work.

One author who guided my journey was Wayne Dyer. His work was the spark that began my journey. I devoured the words in his books and CDs. One phrase he spoke reverberated deep in my soul: "Don't die with the music still in you." I knew each day I had to write so I wouldn't die with the music still in me.

Louise Hay, Esther and Jerry Hicks, Eckhart Tolle, Rhonda Byrne, David Hamilton, Victoria Moran, Lynne McTaggarat, and James O'Donohue—all these authors awakened my spirit so I could find my true self. Michael Beckwith and the Agape International Spiritual Center have taken me to a higher level of consciousness. Thank you so much for live streaming and thanks to all the love streamers. We are family.

Another group of authors supported my alternative views on health, nutrition, physical activity, and weight loss. Their research and conviction to present evidence that challenges the status quo is appreciated. These authors are: Jon Robison, Karen Carrier,

Michael Pollan, Gary Taubes, Christopher Connolly, Hetty Einzig, Linda Bacon, Ph.D., Glenn A. Gaesser, Ph.D., and Paul Campos. I had the good fortune to attend seminars with Jon Robison, author of *The Spirit and Science of Holistic Health*, and Ron Labonte, a passionate health promotion specialist in Canada. They each present their points of view with such passion and conviction, it's contagious. Each of these individuals provided me with insights and the courage of conviction. I hope my work can have the same impact.

Canadians, Paul Liebau, author and Barry Trower, illustrator, captured the essence of living in harmony with yourself and others with a series of small books. The simplicity of each message and image is profound. Thank you so much for allowing me to use your thoughts and illustrations in my book.

Shelly Fuller, you are a kindred spirit. I so appreciate our stimulating conversations, which spawn clarity and move us closer to our destiny. The same is true for you, my dear friend, Karin Perry. Our conversations bring us closer to our true selves. My other dear friends Jeannie and Melissa Hofer have invested time and energy into our friendship. The simplest word or action can offer support and encouragement when embarking on a journey to fulfill a life's dream. Thank you for the simple things you do. You are like family. Theresa Brown, we are also kindred spirits and I so enjoy growing forward with you. Your art is magic.

Steve, Laura, and Tom, my sister's adult children, are great role models for the theories in my book. Every discussion, whether it's about health, medicine or world affairs, is stimulating and reassures me I am on the right track. I wish we could do it more often. Bless your mother to whom this book is dedicated; she was the master of common sense. Laura, a special thank you for advice on the book and for your EFT and TAT interventions. To Tom Sr., my brother-in-law who lives his life with gusto, I thank you for your presence in my life. It mattered more than you will ever know.

Susie Stanley, called me each day and asked me, "How's your book?" I would give her a daily update and then she would reply, "I'm praying for you." It's a beautiful world with you in it, Susie. Andrew Gutormson got me off my writing chair and out walking, insisting I needed to get some exercise. You were right, Andrew. Thank you. Three cheers also to the McDonalds, Huron morning crew for being a great example of positive energy. You're all the best.

It may seem odd to want to thank the town of Huron, my adopted home, but I have been blessed with many opportunities and have always garnered lots of support. I have grown to love the prairie and the friendly nature of the people. It's hard to single out all my treasured friends in Huron, so I can only express my deep gratitude for all the wonderful encounters with each of you. I especially want to thank Peggy Woolridge, my morning walking partner and trusted friend. I figured out a lot of things on our walks.

Then, of course, there are all the people who helped bring the book to life. Thanks to Sammie Justesen, for editing my book in the early stages; you added life and clarity to my words. Your encouragement was a tremendous boost along the way. Marianne Trandall, you are the comma queen and the master proofreader. I can't imagine anyone better. Jane McLaury, your helpful suggestions and endorsement mattered a lot. Kayleen Calkins, and Dan Ryan Dismounts, you are both wonderful graphic artists. What a future you each have ahead of you. Marty Marsh, you're so talented in so many ways. Your imagination is delightful. Thank you so much for your creative touch in producing the Whole Weigh Journal. I sense we will do more things together.

Ariell Ford and Mike Koenings, I want you to know, the Twenty-First Century Book Marketing Seminar was life changing. It was very powerful to be among so many accomplished and aspiring authors, all connected to spirit. Your networks are part of Universal Energy. Thank you for putting me on the right path to success. And finally, thanks to the wonderful people at CreateSpace who made the publishing process easy.

Thank you all for the gifts of your spirit, your words, your friendship, and your being. With the help of each of you, I believe in me. I feel good. Thank you.

About The Author

Over the past thirty years, Charlotte Denny Henley has enjoyed several roles as a fitness trainer, speaker, business owner, and college professor. She served as a community animator for ParticipACTION Ontario, an organization that helps communities increase their citizens' physical activity levels. She is a certified True Colors Personality Facilitator and Certified Wellness Coach, and is trained in the Spirit and Science of Holistic Health. She was awarded a Special Achievement Award from the Province of Ontario for distinguished contribution to the field of fitness and is a former South Dakota Business Woman of the Year. She and her husband Canadian and U.S. College Football Hall of Famer Garney Henley enjoy six grown children between them and live in Huron, South Dakota. *Whole Weigh* is her first book.

Hi I'm Charlotte the author of *Whole Weigh*, the person described above. The description includes all the things I have done in life that make me feel credible in writing this book, but the real me is connected to all of you and no different than you. I am trying to make my way through this life the best way I can, with what I've got at this moment in time. I want to make a difference. I want my life to have value. I want to generate good energy and come from a place of love. I struggle, but I am getting better over time. This book was part of my journey and revealed my personal fears. If you are reading these words, I am so grateful and hope that I was able to inspire you on your journey. Peace and blessings.

Need a Speaker?
Contact Charlotte at charlotte@wholeweigh.com
Get a FREE Whole Weigh Journal at www.wholeweigh.com
Visit Whole Weigh on Facebook for Inspiration.

Printed in Great Britain
by Amazon.co.uk, Ltd.,
Marston Gate.